CURE OR PREVENT DIABETES USING A NOVEL THREE-HOUR POST-MEAL GLUCOSE HOME TESTING PROTOCOL. A REVOLUTIONARY WAY TO NORMALIZE BLOOD SUGARS.

<u>DISCLOSURE</u>

Conflict of interests. Author has no pertinent financial interests with the subject matter, materials discussed, or any web links provided except for an author's book mentioned in the text. Author provides medical advice to veterans as part of his employment. Any nutritional advice given by author in the private sector is free of charge.

Disclaimer. You should consult with your own nutritionally oriented physician or healthcare practitioner, as insulin resistance improvement will require adjusting diabetic prescription medications accordingly. Links to commercial products are for illustrative reasons only.

<u>CONTENTS</u>   PAGE

<u>ABOUT THE AUTHOR</u>

Physician, researcher, and self-taught nutritionist, born in Spain, Manuel Moran, MD, is certified by the American Board of Surgery and by the American Board of Colon and Rectal Surgery. He went to medical school at the University of Salamanca in Spain and obtained a Ph.D. at the same University. He was number 6 out of 16,000 applicants taking the national residency qualification exam in Spain, 1981. After finishing a 5-year General Surgery training at the University Hospital in Salamanca, he did another 5-year General Surgery training at the University of North Dakota in USA. Then he did a one-year fellowship in Colon and Rectal Surgery at the Alton Ochsner Medical Foundation in New Orleans, USA. Clinical Assistant Professor at Texas Tech School of Medicine, Amarillo, TX, 1994-1997, while he was working at the VA Medical Center, he taught many medical students, as well as family practice and general surgery residents.

He has published 26 scientific articles in peer reviewed medical journals and has 28 podium presentations or posters in international meetings as well as two presentations at medical courses and one chapter in a medical book.

While working full-time as a surgeon and acting as the president of Central Minnesota Surgeons, Ltd., he also obtained a law degree (third in his class) at William Mitchell College of Law in Minnesota, USA. He had a limited law practice for a few years but finally decided to focus on Medicine and health prevention, currently working full-time at the VA Medical Center in Saint Cloud, MN and doing endoscopies (colonoscopy, upper endoscopy) in the private sector. The author's mother is also a self-taught nutritionist who had a positive influence allowing him to realize most medical conditions are either preventable or reversible.

While working as a surgeon over the last few decades, it became increasingly frustrating the obvious increase in diabetes, obesity, heart disease, and many other health problems. The lack of preventative support to his patients by the official medical establishment prompted him to write a one-page pamphlet with instructions on how to stay healthy, which he gave to his patients. Later those instructions became two pages, three pages . . . and, finally, a book *Fountain of Health. Regain your Health, Happiness and lose Weight. A revolution in Health for everybody (*in print).

Author has provided free nutritional advice to his patients for many years. Currently, author has designed a randomized study to determine potential beneficial effects of sodium bicarbonate (baking soda) with vitamin D3 for the prevention of viral upper respiratory infections (colds, influenza/flu) and is in the process of opening a functional medicine clinic to prevent or reverse chronic degenerative medical conditions.

The specific interest in diabetes and developing a new method for reversing this disease rose out of two facts. First, official medicine seems to be oblivious to what causes diabetes despite an overwhelming amount of scientific evidence. While interacting with and teaching first year family residents at the VA Medical Center in St. Cloud, USA, he asked five recently finished medical school family practice residents what is the main cause of diabetes. Not even one family practice resident knew the correct answer, which is fat. Every family practice resident asked thought it was carbohydrates or sugar. How can this be possible? How can these future primary care providers help their diabetic patients? Second, despite being completely "healthy", not

CURE OR PREVENT DIABETES

suffering from a single medical condition, and on no medications, one day a screening A1c hemoglobin was abnormal at 5.7, which is the lowest number to make a diagnosis of pre-diabetes. Never let a crisis goes to waist. This became a great opportunity to research this topic and experiment with different ways to improve insulin resistance. The information gained can be shared now with the entire World, for the benefit of everybody.

CURE OR PREVENT DIABETES

<u>INTRODUCTION</u>

Let me be clear. At least in Western countries, people are poisoning themselves with the food they eat. The environmental pollution greatly compounds the problem. Although it may take a few decades for the harmful consequences to manifest themselves, in some cases it can take just a few years. Without good research and understanding of these issues, it will be difficult—if not impossible—to comprehend and benefit from the information provided in this book, which includes scientific information available in the literature as well as my own research.

This book focuses on diabetes, how to prevent it or reverse it. Good health, in general, requires a multi-action approach as described in my book *Fountain of Health. Regain your Health, Happiness and lose Weight. A revolution in Health for everybody,* by Dorrance Publishing.[1]

You can reverse prediabetes or diabetes mostly by avoiding certain fats and testing your body's response to other foods using a 3-hour post-meal home glucose protocol, which I have developed. The earlier the diabetes stage, the easier will be normalizing glucose levels and insulin sensitivity. A few other interventions to normalize insulin resistance should also be considered. Blood glucose level improvement can be achieved in a short time period but normalizing or curing the insulin receptor is more like running a marathon, it is a slow process and it might take months or even years. Normal cell function requires a healthy wall membrane, something most people lack because they eat a high ratio of omega 6 to omega 3 fatty acids. Once a healthy diet is implemented, it takes 9 months for all membrane cells to regenerate. It took many years, sometimes a life-long time, to develop insulin resistance. Perseverance and patience are necessary virtues for those in the process of regaining good health.

When referring to diabetes, this book refers to type 2 diabetes mellitus. Mellitus refers to the sweet taste of urine when glucose is lost in the urine, something that usually requires a blood glucose greater than 200. This was the way diabetes was diagnosed long time ago. Diabetes insipidus is an unusual condition, not related to high blood glucose, you do not have to worry about it. Diabetes, or diabetes mellitus, can be divided in three types but for simplicity we will divide in type 1 and type 2. Type 1 diabetes is an autoimmune disease characterized by lack of insulin production. Pancreatic cells making insulin are damaged and insulin levels drop. Patients need insulin injections to survive. Type 1 diabetic patients do not have insulin resistance. The hallmark of type 2 diabetes insulin resistance (high blood glucose despite high insulin levels). Type 1 diabetes is beyond the scope of this book.

We live in a society where people have become accustomed to being given "a pill" for any illness they suffer. The notion of avoiding what is causing the disease is foreign to many people. Medical providers promptly treat chronic diseases with medications that have side effects and do not cure the underlying cause, a clear recipe for disaster. This approach has led to the skyrocketing of chronic medical conditions, with the associated chronic suffering of a very large percentage of the population, a percentage that continues increasing every decade. People have been conditioned to asking for a quick remedy, "give me a pill", instead of being taught on how to take care of their health by avoiding the harmful behavior. If some food products are damaging your body, forget about "taking a pill" to get better, it WILL NOT work, and the long-term suffering will be unavoidable. People need to take over their health, make the appropriate dietary and lifestyle changes, and use their medical providers to fine tune their good health. It will not be possible to get well or prevent diseases if people persist on harming their bodies with unhealthy foods. Eventually, regenerative technology will become available to rejuvenate the body. Until then, though, you must avoid the offending food or behavior. In an ideal society, primary care providers will be very highly reimbursed to keep their patients healthy. Once a patient develops a chronic medical condition, like diabetes, heart disease, hypertension (high blood pressure), etc., payments for the provider for that patient will be significantly lower. In other words, major emphasis will be placed in keeping people healthy instead of treating sick patients. Of course, this will not be possible until all sources of pollution and toxins, not just unhealthy food, are eliminated.

Diabetes has become a worldwide plague; its prevalence continues increasing without end in sight. It is the leading cause of blindness, kidney failure, lower limb amputations, peripheral neuropathy (leg pain), and so on. It is also a major contributor to heart disease (heart attacks), strokes, erectile dysfunction (impotence), and premature deaths. Expenses related to diabetic care as well as patient suffering are staggering.

Type 2 diabetes is mostly due to insulin resistance although there can be unusual cases (like arsenic toxicity) that can present with decreased insulin production. At least initially, a large amount of insulin is secreted, but cells have become insulin resistant and glucose accumulates in the blood. Too much glucose in the blood causes chronic inflammation and many other adverse effects (like advanced glycation end products – AGEs), which eventually will lead to decreased insulin production in the late stages of the disease. This should be a good reason to take appropriate therapeutic and preventive measures as early as possible, ideally even before somebody develops prediabetes. The notion of PREVENTION is critical, not just when dealing with diabetes but also with all other chronic degenerative conditions, like heart disease, strokes, osteoporosis, dementia, autoimmune diseases, and so on. By the time a diagnosis of prediabetes (even before diabetes) has been made, many persons already have developed diabetic complications. In addition, if no appropriate measures are taken, 75% of people with prediabetes will develop diabetes within ten years.

Type 2 diabetes was also called adult onset diabetes years ago but at this time it affects all generations, including children, and that name has fallen into disuse.

Blood "sugar" is blood glucose, since sugar is a combination of fifty percent glucose and fructose but only glucose is being measured. Blood glucose will be used from now on.

There is nothing like being too young to be worried about diabetes, since even children are developing insulin resistance. Although older people tend to excuse themselves from eating healthy because "it is too late for me", the truth is eating healthy and exercising becomes more important the older the person is.

Part 1 of this book focuses on the 3-hour post-meal glucose testing, which is of critical importance to reverse diabetes. Diabetes can be improved by following several well-known recommendations but without doing the 3-hour post-meal glucose testing is like walking in the dark. It is not possible to predict how a specific fat, food, or meal, will affect a specific person. In addition, the maximum challenge 3-hours post-meal glucose testing is crucial to reverse diabetes because without this test it will not be possible to find out those fats that are harmful only when larger amounts are ingested. Other pertinent knowledge or information will also be discussed.

The role of toxins as the real initial disrupter of the insulin receptor will be discussed in part 2 of the book. Eliminating the offending toxins is going to be the only way to actually "cure" diabetes instead of just reversing it. Reader beware, this is going to be a much longer and time-consuming process. Patience and perseverance will be the key to success.

Part 3 will include author's personal experience improving his insulin sensitivity.

A. REVERSING DIABETES (NORMALIZING INSULIN RESISTANCE)

CHAPTER 1. DIAGNOSIS

A diagnosis of diabetes can be made with several tests that measure blood glucose or glucose related parameters.

1. Hemoglobin A1c (A1c).

A1c, glycated hemoglobin, measures the average blood glucose for the prior three months, thus, it does not have to be done fasting. Fifty percent of its value is based on the average blood glucose over the prior month (the third month), the other 50% measures the first two months. It is used not just to diagnose diabetes but also to monitor diabetes treatment. Normal A1c is up to 5.6. Prediabetes is 5.7 to 6.4. Once it reaches 6.5, a diagnosis of diabetes is made if two consecutive tests remain at this level or higher. The higher the number, the more severe the diabetes is, or in other words, the higher the blood glucose levels have been. Tables can be found correlating A1c numbers to average glucose levels. A formula to calculate the average glucose is 28.7 x A1c - 46.7. Higher A1c correlates well with more diabetic complications, thus, good control is critical. A1c used to be normal up to 5.9 but this level had to be decreased to 5.6 because patients were developing diabetic related complications despite having a "normal" A1c. Unfortunately, normal fasting glucose has not been decreased accordingly.

The lower A1c the better although there can be a small J curve once it drops below 5 (worse prognosis when A1c is very low). This means patients with the lowest A1c have more health problems. It might be due to patients with a very A1c having other medical problems, like malnutrition, advanced malignancies, etc. because in general, lower A1c levels correlate with less chronic conditions, like heart disease.

2. Fasting glucose.

A blood glucose is done on an empty stomach, at least 8 hours without any food intake. Normal fasting glucose is under 100. Unfortunately, this number is too high. It probably should be normal only up to 92. Ideal fasting glucose is 86 or less. Using the official numbers accepted by the medical community, prediabetes is diagnosed when the fasting glucose is between 100 and 125 mg/dl. Higher levels indicate diabetes. Abnormal results should be confirmed with a second measurement or an A1c.

3. Two-hour glucose tolerance test.

This test is not used very often. It is mostly done during pregnancy to diagnose gestational diabetes. With the advent of A1c, this test is usually not performed even though in some studies higher incidence of heart disease has been found with the higher normal levels. A normal test is a 2-hour glucose of < 140 mg/dl. Prediabetes is between 140-199 mg/dl. Diabetes is 200 mg/dl or higher.

4. Fasting insulin level.

This is a very important test that can predict future diabetes many years in advance, way before a diagnosis of prediabetes or diabetes has been performed. Thus, it should be used routinely. Unfortunately, physicians do not use this test as part of their routine armamentarium. Reversing insulin resistance will be much easier when this test becomes abnormal but before prediabetes or diabetes are well established.

A fasting insulin level is done on an empty stomach, at least 10 hours but ideally after at least 12 hours. No agreement has been reached on the ideal fasting insulin level. Lower levels have been correlated with longer life expectancy and, thus, I will not bother specifying the lowest "normal" value. Some experts recommend a fasting insulin level < 5-6 uIU/ml although normal is considered by some as less than 8. Laboratories often call it "normal" all the way up to 23 but this high level is anything but normal. A level higher than 8 indicates some degree of insulin resistance.

Higher insulin levels in animals have correlated with age dependent insulin resistance.[1] Although high insulin levels are caused by insulin resistance, the higher insulin levels could also worsen insulin sensitivity. The study mentioned above stated that "Reduced Circulating Insulin Enhances Insulin Sensitivity in Old Mice and Extends Lifespan".

https://reader.elsevier.com/reader/sd/pii/S2211124717308628?token=87E3BFC58BC06B14A26 D44F61797AE549A7ED223340960265A26ECF2B9997C3E26CE05084C1BE7A2D27E5BD63 3A6C7DB

Lower insulin levels have also correlated with longer life expectancy in human beings. This could explain why in some studies patients on a healthy low carbohydrate diet have longer life expectancies.

A more sophisticated way to diagnose insulin resistance is to use the homeostasis model assessment of insulin resistance (HOMA-IR), which requires drawing a fasting insulin level and a fasting glucose at the same time. It is calculated using this formula: insulin x glucose divided by 405. It uses U.S. standard units; insulin in uIU/ml (pmol/L divided by 6); glucose in mg/dl (mmol/L multiplied by 18). You can use a web based calculator to obtain your HOMA-IR[2] https://www.thebloodcode.com/homa-ir-calculator/

Laboratories might not be able to detect an insulin level < 2 uIU/ml. If insulin is not detectable but the person has a high glucose level, this could indicate type 1 diabetes (insulin deficiency) and prompt medical attention is recommended. Low fasting insulin levels can be caused by eating a low carbohydrate diet, like a ketogenic diet, or by a low-calorie diet. A low fasting insulin is not a concern if blood glucose levels and A1c remain normal.

A healthy HOMA-IR range is 0.5-1.4. Less than one indicates good insulin sensitivity. 1.5-1.9 indicates slight insulin resistance. Above 1.9 is a sign of early insulin resistance. A level of 3 or higher is diagnostic of significant or severe insulin resistance. The higher the number, the worse is the insulin resistance.

CURE OR PREVENT DIABETES

For some time before prediabetes and diabetes have developed, insulin levels have been high. Persistent high insulin levels will remain high for quite a long time. Unfortunately, chronically high glucose levels caused by diabetes are quite proinflammatory. This chronic inflammation slowly but steadily destroys the body, leading to heart attacks, strokes, amputations, blindness, and the list goes on and on. The pancreatic cells making insulin, beta cells, are not immune to this process. In a late stage, beta cells will start dying out and insulin levels will start dropping and become lower than normal. Reversing diabetes at this stage of the game will be very difficult, and other therapeutic measures like multiple episodes of 5-day fasting will be needed and might or might not help. This stage is when diabetic patients will also need insulin injections because their pancreas cannot produce enough insulin to control blood glucose levels.

SUMMARY OF CHAPTER

Diabetes can be diagnosed with different tests, but the most practical approach is using A1c hemoglobin. Two consecutive measurements of 6.5 or higher are diagnostic. This test is also quite useful to monitor glucose control in diabetic patients.

Although not the current standard of care, fasting insulin levels and insulin resistance (HOMA-IR) should be measured and calculated routinely in non-diabetic patients. These results will allow early treatment and reversal of insulin resistance even before prediabetes or diabetes have developed, thus, at a much easier stage.

CHAPTER 2. ETIOLOGY (WHAT CAUSES DIABETES)

Knowledge and clear understanding of what causes diabetes is a total necessity in order to reverse diabetes. I have read many books that deal with reversing and controlling diabetes but do not understand or know what causes diabetes, they focus on carbohydrates instead of fats. Even some world-famous authors have missed this point. I will not speculate on how this is possible. In addition, almost every book fails to consider the role of toxins as the original cause of diabetes.

Regrettably, there are big financial interests at stake, interfering with the dissemination of accurate information. For example, it is undeniable saturated animal fats cause insulin resistance, something beyond reasonable doubt and well established in the scientific literature. But the American Diabetes Association website still recommends eating animal products to diabetic patients, including red meat, and I could not find any information in their website explaining that fat intake causes insulin resistance.

Protein does not cause or prevent diabetes (further comments in chapter 5).

1. FATS (most important)

CURE OR PREVENT DIABETES

The main cause of diabetes is fat intake. Let me repeat this concept to make sure it is clear, FAT INTAKE IS THE MAIN CAUSE OF DIABETES, not sugar or carbohydrates as many people still believe. This is a very difficult concept for many people to comprehend, probably because big financial interests are involved. I did a mini experiment and asked five first-year family practice residents (in training) what causes diabetes. One could guess that a physician who just recently (within one year) finished medical school will know perfectly well what causes one of the most devastating diseases, since scientific evidence has been available for close to twenty years. One family practice resident answered "insulin resistance" as the cause of diabetes. This is like saying that the White House is white. Type 2 diabetes and insulin resistance are synonymous. Thus, I had to clarify this point and repeat the question. All five family practice residents stated "carbohydrates" or "sugar" caused diabetes. None was aware of fat (intracellular lipids on the membrane) as the real cause of diabetes. These will be the primary care providers that will be taking care of you in a few years. Hopefully by then this information will be widely available.

Unhealthy fats should always be avoided, no exceptions to this rule. Unfortunately, even healthy fats can increase insulin resistance when handled inappropriately, like high temperature cooking, rancid, or some oils when exposed to light. Sesame oil is also room temperature sensitive and should be stored in the refrigerator.

It was about one century ago, in the early 20th century, when it was found diabetes risk increased with high fat animal diets compared to carbohydrates. At that time, most carbohydrates in the diet were not refined like happens today. This was a clinical observation and did not explain how insulin resistance was caused by fat intake.

We must wait until 2004 for the scientific proof on how insulin resistance occurs. One article in the New England Journal of Medicine showed lipid (fat) deposits inside the cell membrane blocked the insulin receptor, thus causing insulin resistance. [1]

Since then, highly sophisticated MRI technology has allowed researches to demonstrate how fat entering the cells causes diabetes. Many studies have confirmed the original New England Journal of Medicine article. With insulin resistance, higher levels of fat are found in the blood. Intravenous injections of fat cause insulin resistance. When this extra-fat is removed from the blood, insulin resistance subsides. The process is slower when fat is ingested. Fat must be absorbed, and fat blood levels must increase to a certain point. It takes 2.5 to 3 hours for a fatty meal to produce or worsen insulin resistance. I have done many hundreds or thousands of glucose tests on myself and never found any insulin resistance at two hours after fatty intake. This information allows the development and practical use of the 3-hours post-meal glucose testing protocol. A traditional 2-hour post meal glucose test does not provide information on whether a meal is causing insulin resistance.

1.1. UNHEALTHY FATS

Some fats are very unhealthy and should NOT be eating at all. Yes, they contribute to diabetes, but they are so unhealthy that even persons without any insulin resistance should not be eating them.

CURE OR PREVENT DIABETES

Which ones are the unhealthiest fats? The answer is simple, those fats or oils that are man-made. Artificial oils and fats do not exist in nature, the body cannot completely metabolize them. Whatever amount of oil or fat is not metabolized, will create chronic inflammation, arterial deposits (e.g., heart disease, strokes), and insulin resistance.

1.1.1. PROCESSED VEGETABLE OILS. All processed vegetable oils are unhealthy, including canola, corn, cottonseed, safflower, sunflower, and soybean oils. These oils have been processed commercially in multiple unhealthy ways, including chemicals and high temperatures. The exact details of the manufacturing process are beyond the scope of this book, but this information is easily available on the Internet.

There is ample evidence of a direct correlation between the consumption of these oils and the risk of developing diabetes. The industry has falsely labeled these oils as healthy because they "decrease cholesterol" when they are proinflammatory and quite unhealthy. Regardless of how they affect cholesterol levels, these oils are very harmful, increasing not just diabetes but also vascular diseases, like strokes and heart attacks. In addition to their unhealthy nature, they are loaded with omega 6 fatty acids which unbalance the healthy 1:1 omega 6 to omega 3 fatty acid ratio.

Peanut oil is not as unhealthy as the previously mentioned processed vegetable oils but should be avoided. Peanuts are not actual nuts but a legume that has lectins (unhealthy protein), which also come with the oil. Lectins can cause many health conditions, including autoimmune problems.

1.1.2. TRANS FATS. Trans fats, which are partially hydrogenated oils, are extremely unhealthy and should not be consumed at all. Current legislation allows food manufacturers to claim no trans fats if a serving has less than 0.5 grams per serving. Unfortunately, if the serving is relatively small, you may end up eating a significant amount of trans fats. If the label has any "hydrogenated oil" as an ingredient, do not eat it because it has trans fats. This type of fat, if man-made, should be illegal and completely avoided. There is no "safe" amount of trans fat consumption. A small amount of trans fats can be produced during cooking, but these seem to be less harmful. Nevertheless, remember to always cook at low temperatures, as low as possible.

1.1.3. INTERESTERIFIED FATS. From a diabetes point of view, the worse fats are interesterified fats. They have been used by the food industry as an inexpensive alternative to partially hydrogenated oils. For the food industry these fats have several advantages, including longer shelve life and a different melting point, and are included in a large variety of processed foods.

One study found the highest risk of developing insulin resistance was due to this type of fat. Because there is no specific pertinent legislation, the food industry does not have to warn consumers in the label whether this fat is one of the ingredients. The only way to avoid consumption of this fat is by completely avoiding processed food (except single ingredients). This is very important. The insulin receptor will not improve if it remains continuously under attack. Thus, avoiding processed foods is a must.

1.2. SATURATED ANIMAL FATS.

CURE OR PREVENT DIABETES

These fats are in the twilight zone of medical care. Let me explain. Study after study, starting with the many decade long Framingham Heart Study done more than half a century ago, have proven beyond reasonable doubt that saturated animal fats do not cause heart disease. A word of caution, though. For unknown reasons to me, very smart researchers and authors have quickly extrapolated this knowledge and concluded saturated animal fats are safe to eat, with complete disregard to a major body of evidence showing they increase diabetes. It is hard to explain how very intelligent physicians and authors have failed keeping these two issues separate, which has led to confusion among many people.

A large body of medical literature has focused on saturated fats as the main culprit causing diabetes. Several references follow to make sure this point is not arguable. The main conclusions summarized by this author are in bold letters:

1. Petersen KF, et al. Impaired mitochondrial activity in the insulin-resistant offspring of patients with type 2 diabetes. *N Engl J Med.* 2004 Feb 12; 350(7):664-71. **(Intracellular fat blocks the insulin receptor)**

2. Sweeney S. Dietary factors that influence the dextrose tolerance test. A preliminary study. *Arch Intern Med* 1927; 40(6): 818-830. **(Saturated animal fat causes insulin resistance)**

3. Krssak M, et al. Intramyocellular lipid concentrations are correlated with insulin sensitivity in humans: a 1H NMR spectroscopy study. *Diabetology* 1999; 42: 113-116. **(Diabetes caused specifically by saturated fats)**

4. Roden M, et al. Mechanism of Free Fatty Acid-induced insulin Resistance in Humans. *J. Clin. Invest.* 1996; 97: 2859-2865. **(Saturated animal fat causes insulin resistance)**

5. Roden M, Krssak M, Stingl H, et al. Rapid Impairment of Skeletal Muscle Glucose Transport/Phosphorylation by Free Fatty Acids in Humans. *Diabetes* 1999; 48(2): 358-364. **(Saturated animal fat causes insulin resistance)**

6. Lee S, et al. Effects of an overnight lipid infusion on intramyocellular lipid content and insulin sensitivity in African-American versus Caucasian adolescents. *Metabolism Clinical and Experimental* 2013; 62: 417-423. **(Saturated animal fat causes insulin resistance)**

7. Santomauro A TMG. Overnight Lowering of Free Fatty Acids With Acipimox Improves Insulin Resistance and Glucose Tolerance in Obese Diabetic and Nondiabetic Subjects. *Diabetes* 1999; 48(9): 1836-41. **(Saturated animal fat causes insulin resistance)**

8. Roden M. How Free Fatty Acids Inhibit Glucose Utilization in Human Skeletal Muscle. *News Physiol Sci* 2004; 19: 92-96. **(Spillover effect linking obesity to type 2 diabetes)**

9. Bachmann OP, et al. Effects of Intravenous and Dietary Lipid Challenge on Intramyocellular Lipid Content and the Relation With Insulin Sensitivity in Humans. *Diabetes* 2001; 50: 2579-2584. **(Spillover effect linking obesity to type 2 diabetes)**

10. Samuel VT, et al. Mechanisms for Insulin Resistance: Common Threads and Missing Links. *Cell* 148, March 2, 2012. **(Saturated fat raises blood glucose)**

11. Rachek LI. Free Fatty Acids and Skeletal Muscle Insulin Resistance. *Progress in Molecular Biology and Translational Science*, Volume 121. **(Insulin resistance caused by saturated fats, not by unsaturated fats)**

12. Evans WJ. Oxygen-Carrying Proteins in Meat and Risk of Diabetes Mellitus. *JAMA Intern Med* 2013; 173(14): 1335-1336. **(Saturated fats cause insulin resistance)**

13. Perseghin G, et al. Intramyocellular Triglyceride Content Is a Determinant of in Vivo Insulin Resistance in Humans. *Diabetes* Vol 48, August 1999. **(Saturated fat build-up in muscles causes insulin resistance)**

14. Nolan CJ, et al. Lipotoxicity: Why do saturated fatty acids cause and monounsaturated protect against it? *Journal of Gastroenterology and Hepatology* 2009; 24: 703-711. **(Saturated fats cause lipotoxicity)**

15. Ye J. Role of Insulin in the Pathogenesis of Free Fatty Acid-Induced Insulin Resistance in Skeletal Muscle. *Endocrine, Metabolic & Immune Disorders – Drug Targets* 2007; 7: 65-74. **(Insulin creates free fatty acid insulin resistance).**

16. Estadella D, et al. Lipotoxicity: Effects of Dietary Saturated and Transfatty Acids. *Mediators of Inflammation* 2013; article ID 13. **(Saturated and trans fatty acids cause insulin resistance)**

17. Vessby B, et al. Substituting dietary saturated for monounsaturated fat impairs insulin sensitivity in healthy men and women: The KANWU study. *Diabetologia* 2001; 44: 312-319. **(Insulin sensitivity improved by switching from saturated fats to plant fats: insulin sensitivity was impaired on saturated fat but not on monounsaturated fatty acid diet—olive fat)**

18. Martins AR, et al. Mechanisms underlying skeletal muscle insulin resistance induced by fatty acids: importance of the mitochondrial function. *Lipids in Health and Disease* 2012; 11: 30. **(Saturated fats cause insulin resistance—e.g., palmitic acid and stearic acid are potent inducers of insulin resistance → also inhibit key mitochondrial enzymes)**

19. Karlic H., et al. Vegetarian Diet Affects Genes of Oxidative Metabolism and Collagen Synthesis. *Annals of Nutrition & Metabolism* 2008; 53: 29-32. **(On a vegetarian diet have 60% higher expression of fat burning enzyme)**

20. Goff LM, et al. Veganism and its relationship with insulin resistance and intramyocellular lipid. *European Journal of Clinical Nutrition* 2005; 59: 291-298. **(Vegans had lower systolic blood pressure, higher intake of carbohydrates; vegans had less fat in muscle despite having same BMIs)**

21. Gojda J, et al. Higher insulin sensitivity in vegans is not associated with higher mitochondrial density. *European Journal of Clinical Nutrition* 2013; 1310-1315. **(Vegans had better insulin sensitivity, better blood glucose levels, better insulin levels, and higher insulin glucose disposal, as well as improve beta cell function. Thus, veganism is cardioprotective and possibly beta cell protective)**

22. West KM, et al. Influence of Nutritional Factors on Prevalence of Diabetes. *Diabetes* 1971; 20: 99-108, February. **(Animal fat consumption was positively associated with diabetes prevalence)**

23. Snowdon DA, et al. Does a Vegetarian Diet Reduce the Occurrence of Diabetes? *Am J Public Health* 1985; 75: 507-512. **(Eating meat one or more day a week increases the risk of diabetes; risk increases with increased number of days meat was eaten, despite controlling for weight; lower prevalence of diabetes among vegetarians)**

24. Tonstad S, et al. Vegetarian diets and incidence of diabetes in the Adventist Health Study-2. *Nutrition, Metabolism & Cardiovascular Diseases* 2013; 23: 292-299. **(Diabetes decreases with the level of vegetarian diet: 0.22 for vegans, 0.39 for lactoovovegetarian, 0.49 for pescovegetarian, 0.72 for semivegetarian. N = 89,224 individuals. Same is applicable to high blood pressure and BMI)**

25. Chiu THT, et al.   Taiwanese Vegetarians and Omnivores: Dietary Composition, Prevalence of Diabetes and IFG. *PLoS* 2014 February 11; 9(2): e88547. **(Vegetarian compared to traditional Asian diet with a very small amount of animal products (women ate a single serving per week, men every few days): men eating vegetarian had half the rate—0.49—of diabetes and 0.66 for IFG; in pre-menopausal women: diabetes 0.26 and IFG 0.60; and in menopausal women: diabetes 0.25 and IFG 0.73. IFG = pre-diabetes = impaired fasting glucose. No analysis done between vegetarian and vegan but there were no cases of diabetes among vegans)**

26. Cunha DA, et al. Death Protein 5 and p53-Upregulated Modulator of Apoptosis Mediate the Endoplasmic Reticulum Stress—Mitochondrial Dialog Triggering Lipotoxic Rodent and Human beta cell Apoptosis. *Diabetes* 2012; 61: 2763-2775. **(Mostly saturated fat (palmitate) negatively affects beta cells; olives, nuts and avocados (oleate) has a minimally negative effect)**

27. Xiao C, et al. Differential effects of monounsaturated, polyunsaturated and saturated fat ingestion on glucose-stimulated insulin secretion, sensitivity and clearance in overweight and obese, non-diabetic humans.*Diabetologia* 2006; 49: 1371-1379. **(Saturated fat negatively affects insulin secretion and function; increased insulin resistance and decreased insulin production within hours of saturated fat ingestion)**

28. Evans WJ. Oxygen-Carrying Proteins in Meat and Risk of Diabetes Mellitus. *JAMA Intern* Med 2013; 173 (14): 1335-1336. **(Red meat consumption increases diabetes risk)**

29. Cao J, Feng XX, Yang NB, et al. Saturated Free Fatty Acid Sodium Palmitate-Induced Lipoapoptosis by Targeting Glycogen Synthase Kinase-3B Activation in Human Liver Cells. *Dig Dis Sci* 2014; February 59(2): 346-57 **(Fat—e.g., palmitate-- in meat and dairy are universally toxic; fat in nuts and avocados (monounsaturated fatty acids—MUFA—e.g., oleat—are not toxic)**

30. Parker DR, et al. Relationship of dietary saturated fatty acids and body habitus to serum insulin concentrations: the Normative Aging Study. *Am J Clin Nutr* 1993; 58: 129-36. **(Obesity and saturated fat intake increase fasting and postprandrial insulin concentrations)**

31. Maron DJ. Saturated Fat Intake and Insulin Resistance in Men With Coronary Artery Disease. *Circulation* 1991; 84: 2020-2027. **(Saturated fat as a contributor to insulin resistance)**

32. Wang L, et al. Plasma fatty acid composition and incidence of diabetes in middle-aged adults: the Atherosclerosis Risk in Communities (ARIC) Study. *Am J Clin Nutr* 2003; 78: 91-8. **(Increased plasma saturated fatty acids worsened the risk of diabetes)**

33. Taylor R. Pathogenesis of type 2 diabetes: tracing the reverse route from cure to cause. *Diabetologia* 2008; 51: 1781-1789. **(Diabetes is caused by the consumption of too many calories rich in saturated fats in the setting of unfavorable genetic background)**

34. Feskens EJ, Sluik D, and Woudenbergh GJ. Meat Consumption, Diabetes, and Its Complications. *Curr Diab Rep* 2013 April; 13(2): 298-306. **(Diabetes risk increased with meat consumption, worse with processed meat and partially for processed poultry)**

35. Palli BB, et al. Association between dietary meat consumption and incident type 2 diabetes: the EPIC-InterAct study. The InterAct Consortium. *Diabetologia* 2013; 56: 47-59. **(Meat consumption increased risk of diabetes; also seen an increase risk of diabetes among workers in the meat industry, unclear cause)**

36. Zoncu R, et al. mTor: from growth signal integration to cancer, diabetes and ageing. *Nature Reviews Molecular Biology* January 2011; volume 12. **(Excessive animal/dairy protein/food consumption over stimulates mTor and may increase diabetes due to increase intake of leucine)**

37. Liu G, et al. Meat Cooking Methods and Risk of Type 2 Diabetes: Results From Three Prospective Cohort Studies. *Diabetes Care* 2018 Mar; dc171992. **(More diabetes among those cooking their meals at higher temperatures)**

Based on the many studies mentioned above, saturated animal fats cause diabetes, this fact is by now well established and not questionable. Specific studies have shown red meat increases diabetes. You can draw your own conclusions on why some medical associations and societies do not acknowledge this evidence and fail to warn diabetic patients accordingly.

Although saturated fats are more heat stable than other fats or oils, they are still heat sensitive as referenced above.[37] A fascinating question is whether never heated saturated fats cause diabetes. We do not have a final answer to this question. Further research will be needed. I think it is likely that non-heated animal fats do not cause insulin resistance.

I personally did several 3-hour post-meal glucose tests after eating four or six raw egg yolks in addition to a regular meal and experienced absolutely no insulin resistance (3-hour glucose around 100). On the other hand, after eating four very soft-boiled yolks (with the yolk still mostly liquid) on several occasions, I noticed a significant 3-hour insulin resistance (3-hour glucose around 140). How the food industry processes fat is important. For example, ghee (clarified butter) is heated during the manufacturing process. Whether the heating was enough for some person to develop some insulin resistance is something difficult to predict, thus the need to do the 3-hour post-meal glucose testing.

The members of the Maasai tribe of Kenya and Tanzania do not suffer from heart disease or diabetes despite eating a diet with 66% of calories from animal fat (33-45% of their caloric intake is saturated animal fat). But a large percentage of those animal fat calories come from drinking 3-5 quarts (about 3-5 liters) of raw milk per day. This is further evidence that saturated animal fats might not cause diabetes if not heated. Of course, it must be disclosed that other factors might be in play. For example, the Maasai do not eat any processed food or refined carbohydrates. They also have much less exposure to modern pollutants, chemical, and toxins.

1. 3. HEALTHY FATS THAT BECOME UNHEALTHY

Healthy fats in reasonable amounts and not heated do not cause insulin resistance. In moderate amounts, some healthy unheated fats even decrease the risk of diabetes. Healthy oils include organic coconut oil, extra virgin olive oil, omega 3 oil (fish and cod liver oil) of a high-quality source, avocado oil, macadamia oil, walnut oil, sesame seed oil, and flax seed oil. Any of these oils is unhealthy once it has been heated enough or if it has been refined. Thus, stay away from any type of refined olive oil (sometimes refined and extra virgin are mixed).

Some oils have been found to have protective effect against diabetes, like olive oil and nuts oil. I still would caution against eating a very large amount just in case, although some people might be able to get away with it.

Omega 3 fish oil may decrease diabetes risk, but it is temperature sensitive. Never buy inexpensive fish oil capsules because you will not know what manufacturing temperature was used. Some experts have advised curing salmon instead of cooking it, which can be done in the refrigerator. Eskimo diet is high in fat (omega 3 from fish oil) and their diabetes prevalence is significantly lower (3.3% vs. 7.7%).[38] Eskimos ate much more fish oil than what is consumed in the 48 lower states. Although 70% were obese or overweight, diabetes prevalence was low at 3.3%.

Unfortunately, every oil will become unhealthy when heated enough or when it becomes rancid. Some oils are light sensitive. Thus, try to keep fresh oil in your house and do not heat it or at least do not heat much. It is a shame when people buy expensive oil, like extra virgin olive oil, and then they use it in the frying pan at high temperatures.

A major unknown issue when heating oils, is up to what temperature is it safe. Oils have different and quite variable smoke points. The same might be applicable to a maximum safe temperature. Unfortunately, it is not known at what specific temperatures oils start becoming unhealthy, and thus start increasing insulin resistance.

Reheating oil degrades it even further and should be always avoided. Once used, reusing or reheating the oil will make it unhealthy and will increase the risk of developing diabetes.

1.4. SATURATED PLANT-BASED FAT (COCONUT OIL).

Coconut oil is a saturated fat and, thus, the most heat resistant oil. This is the reason why some people advise the use of coconut oil for cooking. In some studies, coconut oil has been found to decrease the risk of diabetes.

When reading the fine print of studies stating diabetes is caused by saturated fats, it becomes apparent the researchers were only studying saturated animal fats, not saturated plant-based fats like coconut oil. Unfortunately, the information about saturated animal fats has been extrapolated by many to saturated plant-based fats. Few animal and human studies have been performed with coconut oil. So far, no evidence is available to blame coconut oil. In fact, in some studies coconut oil has been shown to decrease the risk of diabetes. The explanation can be simple. Although coconut oil is mostly saturated fat, the molecular arrangement is different than the one found in the animal world.

In addition, epidemiological evidence should be considered, and it is certainly favorable to coconut oil. Until a few decades ago, coconut oil was the main oil consumed in Sri Lanka without any apparent side effects. The same can be said about the Pacific Islanders and some parts of India. Nevertheless, when consumption of processed vegetable oils increased, so did chronic degenerative conditions like diabetes and heart disease. Very impressive data comes from the Tokelau Island, somewhere between Hawaii and Australia. 54-62% of calories eaten by the Atoll people are from coconut. 53% of their caloric intake is from fat, 48 being saturated fat. But the Atoll people do not suffer from diabetes, heart disease, or obesity.

In general, animal fats are much more heat stable than oils, something critical when deciding what to cook with and at what temperatures. Coconut oil has the same advantage, it is much more heat stable compared to other oils, like olive, or avocado oils. In fact, some oils are so heat-unstable that should not be used for cooking (e.g., flax seed oil, omega 3 oils, etc.).

2. EPIGENETICS

Obviously, genetic predisposition also plays a role. Epigenetics is a very important concept. It refers to the interaction of genetic predisposition with environmental factors. The good news is most people will not develop diabetes if they stay away from the triggering environmental factors. A positive family history for diabetes should be a good motivation to take precautionary measures.

3. COOKING TEMPERATURE

Another interesting twist in the etiology of diabetes is cooking temperature. We also have evidence showing that the same amount of animal fats will cause more diabetes when the food is cooked at the highest temperatures despite eating the same meals.[37]

As previously mentioned, it is not known whether saturated animal fats might not cause diabetes if they were never heated. My 3-hour post-meal glucose testing after eating 4-6 raw egg yolks indicates that maybe never heated animal fats do not cause diabetes. Further research is needed.

I have personally done home-made milk chocolate with a melanger (stone grinder) using the same ingredients but found insulin resistance only when chocolate was ground at a higher temperature (140 degrees Fahrenheit vs. 100 degrees) for 24 hours. This indicates how important is cooking at low temperatures.

For this reason, how the food industry processes fats is of critical importance. For example, ghee (clarified butter) in heated during the manufacturing process. Whether this low heat is enough for some persons to develop some insulin resistance is difficult to predict, thus the need to do the 3-hour post-meal glucose testing.

Unhealthy fats, mentioned above, should be avoided even if not heated at home. Moreover, unhealthy fats become more harmful when heated or reheated. The higher the cooking temperature, the more harmful they become. The more times oil is reheated, the more harmful it becomes. By the time oil reaches its smoke point, it is such a highly toxic product that needs to be thrown away.

The most heat-stable fats are saturated fats, both animal and plant based. Consider this fact when cooking.

CURE OR PREVENT DIABETES

Ideally, oils should not be heated, maybe except for coconut oil, but a 3-hours post-meal testing is still needed.

4. OBESITY

The number of adipose (fat) cells (adipocytes) is well established and stable in adults. In other words, when people become obese the number of adipocytes remains the same. Cells just accumulate more fat. Unfortunately, this has a quite detrimental effect on diabetes. The pressure inside the adipose cells increases too much and lipids (fat) leaks out the cells into the blood stream. Increased fat in the blood is well known to cause insulin resistance. With worsening obesity, insulin resistance becomes more pronounced, leading to a vicious cycle. The body releases more insulin to deal with increased glucose levels in the blood. Higher insulin levels lock fat calories in the cells, not making those calories available to the body. This is the reason why fasting has worked well in severe obesity as well as in obese diabetics, because it breaks this vicious cycle.

At this time, it is well accepted by the medical community that obesity is an independent factor causing diabetes. Nevertheless, this "truth" has been challenged by toxic analyses as it will be discussed later.

5. OTHER CONTRIBUTING FACTORS

5.1. Excess refined carbohydrates

Fructose in large amounts becomes a metabolic poison because the body is not designed to process it. It is well accepted that sugary drinks, like soda with high fructose corn syrup, increase the risk of diabetes. Carbohydrates do not directly interfere with the insulin receptor. But a large amount of sugar, which is half fructose, can lead to fatty liver disease and increased blood lipids. Fatty liver disease causes liver insulin resistance. Increased blood lipids cause insulin resistance in muscle cells. We are not talking of the carbohydrates that come in whole foods. It would very difficult—if possible—to overdue consumption of those carbohydrates. For example, most people will eat one apple, not five or six apples. The problem starts when food is processed and somebody decides that if one apple is healthy, they will drink the juice of several apples. Here the fructose load becomes harmful to the body. Sugary drinks should be completely avoided, including fruit juices.

As a rule of thumb, complex carbohydrates like the ones found in whole foods, are safe to eat. Refined carbohydrates cause chronic inflammation and should be avoided. Chronic inflammation is the root cause of most modern chronic degenerative diseases, like heart disease. High triglycerides are a significant risk factor for heart disease but can be easily normalize by avoiding refined carbohydrates. Also avoid unhealthy fats.

A good example to support the safety of eating complex carbohydrates is the Tukisenta in Papua New Guinea (an island north of Australia). More than 90% of their caloric intake comes from many varieties of sweet potatoes. Carbohydrates represent 94.6% of their caloric intake but they do not have any diabetes, obesity, or hypertension (high blood pressure). And heart disease is rare.

Ideally, people should eat a large amount of above the ground vegetables and some fruits (best if organic and grown locally).

5.2. Excess calories.

This etiologic (causing) factor has not been studied as well as fats but seems to be a contributory factor. Excess calories, as described as more food consumed that needed, increases oxygen free radicals. Some free radicals are unavoidable. In fact, they play a role in normal cell function. But too many free radicals speed up the aging process. Excess calorie intake is not the main cause of diabetes, but it would be prudent to avoid it when trying to reverse insulin resistance. Besides accelerating aging, excess calories could lead to obesity, a contributing factor to develop diabetes.

5.3. Lack of physical exercise.

Physical exercise alone has not been able to fight obesity because the number of calories burned is way too small and not too significant compared to multiple other factors involved in obesity. Nevertheless, physical exercise is quite helpful for improving insulin resistance because it increases the number of mitochondria in the muscle cells. Mitochondria are the energy generators inside the cells. Nothing works or survives well without adequate energy. Exercise is very effective in increasing the number of mitochondria. This increase in energy production greatly benefits the insulin receptor. Several supplements will increase the number of mitochondria, but nothing works as well as good physical exercise, like high intensity interval training. Moreover, those supplements are expensive. In short, avoid sedentary life.

5.4. Toxins (accepted explanation by current official Medicine)

Some scientific evidence in peer reviewed medical journals has correlated diabetes with environmental toxins, like heavy metals and organic pollutants.[39, 40] Organic pollutants and heavy metals are contributors not just to diabetes but also to obesity. Interestingly, the main source of organic pollutants is the intake of dietary animal fats.[40] This fact would be another reason to eat mostly a plant-based diet.

Thus, official Medicine accepts that toxins play some role in diabetes. It would not be surprising if official Medicine acknowledged toxins as the major cause of diabetes in the near future. So far, more than 400 studies have found some relationship between heavy metals and diabetes.[41]

Aluminum is highly neurotoxic and causes autism and dementia. It crosses the intestinal barrier (lining of the gut) when combined with glyphosate (the main ingredient in RoundUp[R]) which comes with GMO foods. Aluminum also has been found to worsen fasting blood glucose and increase diabetes risk.[42]

Even considering official Medicine only, enough evidence is available to recommend routine detoxification for anybody with insulin resistance.

5.5. Chronically elevated blood insulin levels.

Some authors think chronically elevated insulin levels cause insulin resistance. The explanation some famous authors have given is that the insulin receptor becomes desensitize when exposed to chronically elevated insulin levels. Thus, some of those authors blame diabetes to the consumption of large amounts of carbohydrates. For unclear reasons to me, most people have been sold-out to this idea. It is true that this mechanism does happen in other circumstances, like tolerance (less effective) to narcotics when used for a while. But this mechanism is certainly not the main cause of diabetes. Carbohydrates will spike blood glucose, but this does not directly affect the insulin receptor.

Nevertheless, at least one animal study showed rats with higher insulin levels did have worse insulin sensitivity.[43] It is certainly possible that chronically elevated high insulin levels worsen insulin sensitivity, although high insulin was not what caused insulin resistance in the beginning. In addition, nobody will disagree that chronically elevated insulin levels cause chronic inflammation, which can eventually harm the pancreatic insulin producing beta cells. This would be a late stage of diabetes and would lead to low blood insulin levels, though.

In any case, this would be another good reason to include fasting as part of the armamentarium for diabetes reversal.

6. TOXINS, TOXINS, TOXINS. THE REAL CULPRIT CAUSING INSULIN RECEPTOR DAMAGE (NON-OFFICIAL EXPLANATION).

This information leads to a logical conclusion. Prevention or detoxification of toxins will be an integral part of diabetes management and will be discussed later, in Part 2 of the book.

SUMMARY OF CHAPTER

Fat is the main immediate cause of insulin resistance. Saturated animal fats are the best studied contributor to diabetes, as shown in many scientific studies. But all unhealthy fats are implicated and should be avoided, including all man-made oils and fats (processed vegetable oils, trans fats, margarines, and interesterified oils). Heating fats increases the harmful effect of fats or oils on the insulin receptor. The higher the temperature, the more harmful the effect is. Even healthy fats will cause insulin resistance if heated enough or altered in any way (e.g., rancid, exposed to oxygen and light).

Coconut oil (saturated plant-based fat) does not cause diabetes and might have protective effect.

Avoiding offending fats will reverse diabetes and normalize blood glucose but it will not cure the defective insulin receptor. The reason is simple. Food and environmental toxins must damage the insulin receptor first. The implications are very significant. To prevent or cure diabetes, harmful toxins must be avoided or detoxified.

CHAPTER 3. PROBLEM WITH (A) MEDICATIONS THAT INCREASE INSULIN OR WITH (B) INSULIN SUPPLEMENTATION

This issue is rather critical because many diabetic patients are still being treated with medications that have harmful long-term consequences.

It is beyond the scope of this book to discuss worse patient cardiovascular mortality (death rate) when diabetic patients are started on oral medications that increase insulin production or, even worse, on insulin injections. Examples of this type of oral antidiabetic medications include sulfonylureas (e.g., glyburide, glimepiride) and meglitinides (nateglinide, repaglinide). This would not be applicable to those medications that do not increase insulin levels, like metformin which enhances the effect of insulin instead.[1]

Intensive glucose control in acutely ill patients, like after major surgeries or in the Intensive Care Unit, has been studied. Tightly controlled blood glucose increased complications and mortality. Despite good scientific evidence available, many experts do not understand this issue. Just as an example, Goldman et al. published an article titled "Effect of Intensive Glycemic Control on Risk of Lower Extremity Amputation" in 2018. [2] The authors concluded in the abstract "ICG (intensive glucose control) was associated with a reduction in the risk of LEA (lower extremity amputation)." Their abstract does not mention this trial was discontinued by the pharmaceutical sponsor after an average of 3.7 years of follow up because there was a significant increase in deaths in the intensive glucose control group.

Increased insulin levels are pro-inflammatory. In other words, higher insulin levels cause chronic inflammation, which is the main cause of all modern degenerative diseases, like heart attacks, strokes, dementia, and so on. In addition, insulin is an anabolic hormone. In other words, it increases body weight by adding more adipose tissue (fat), and it locks the calories in fat, which is out-of-reach of the body's caloric needs. Increased weight worsens diabetes, in fact, obesity is officially considered an independent contributing factor. Once a patient is started on insulin injections, in addition to oral diabetes medications, gaining extra weight becomes almost inevitable. This creates a very difficult-to-break vicious cycle, life becomes an uphill battle with not much hope in sight. Everything should be done to avoid reaching this stage.

Diabetes management or reversal should be focused on improving insulin sensitivity, not on increasing circulating insulin levels which mask the disease (lower blood glucose) but has significant harmful side effects.

SUMMARY OF CHAPTER

High insulin levels are very unhealthy. Increased insulin levels do happen in patients taking insulin injections or the type of oral diabetic medications that increase insulin production. Chronic higher insulin levels correlate with worse survival. Thus, glucose control should be based on improving insulin resistance, not on increasing blood insulin levels.

CHAPTER 4. 3-HOUR POST-MEAL HOME GLUCOSE TESTING.

1. THE 3-HOUR POST-MEAL HOME GLUCOSE TESTING FOR REGULAR MEALS.

The scientific basis for this test is very simple. I have described it in a medical journal[1]

The main reason for the insulin receptor to become insensitive to circulating insulin in the blood is lipid (fat) deposits inside the cell membrane. After a meal, fat must be digested, absorbed, and enter the muscle cells. It takes about 2.5 to 3 hours for a meal containing fat to produce insulin resistance. Fat is metabolized slower than protein or carbohydrates. Thus, the 2-hour post-meal blood glucose performed by the medical community will completely miss the diagnosis for two reasons: (a) it is not enough time to produce affect the insulin receptor, and (b) the test can done with liquid glucose instead of a real meal. I have done many hundreds of 2-hour and 3-hour post meal glucose tests and the 2-hour one always fails to detect insulin resistance caused by that meal.

Nevertheless, the 3-hour glucose testing still needs a 2-hour blood glucose so that both glucose results can be compared. After eating a regular meal, a blood glucose spike will happen within the first 60 minutes after the end of the meal. How quickly this spike happens greatly depends on the amount and type of carbohydrates ingested. A meal with refined carbohydrates could spike glucose within 20-30 minutes. Complex carbohydrates, likes the ones in vegetables, will take much longer. Carbohydrates in food will spike glucose relatively rapidly, within one hour, despite coming with fiber. In any case, the 2-hour post-meal blood glucose should be decreasing and usually will be lower than the 1-hour glucose. Thus, the 3-hour post-meal blood glucose should be similar or lower than the 2-hour glucose. An exception could be a very large meal that takes a few hours to be digested. This could be the case when somebody is eating only one meal per day. In this case, the 3-hour post-meal blood glucose could be similar or somewhat higher than the 2-hour glucose even in the absence of insulin resistance. To keep things simple, we will consider the 3-hour post-meal blood glucose to be abnormal if it is more than 10% larger than the 2-hour glucose. This is an arbitrary threshold and future research might come up with a different percentage. If in doubt, the solution is simple. Eat the same amount and type of fat on a different day but significantly decrease total calories consumed if the number of calories was large the first time. Also decrease some the amount of foods rich in fiber, since it will be digested and absorbed over a longer period of time.

At least initially, my advice is to perform a 1-hour, 2-hour, and 3-hour post meal glucose testing. The 1-hour glucose can provide useful information, also. An ideal diet is one that does not spike much blood glucose. The higher the glucose spike, the unhealthier the meal was. Until insulin resistance has normalized, carbohydrates need to be minimized to prevent or minimize a post meal glucose spike. The 1-hour post meal glucose will allow determining how to modify or decrease carbohydrate intake to maintain a relatively stable glucose curve, without any major spikes. Once a person has normal insulin sensitivity, the amount of carbohydrates can be increased as determined by the 1-hour glucose results.

What to do if the 3-hour post-meal is significantly larger than the 2-hour glucose? In this case, a 4-hour post-meal blood glucose is needed. If the 4-hour glucose is higher than the 3-hour glucose, keep on doing hourly blood glucose levels until a blood glucose is less than the prior one. How long it takes for the blood glucose to start coming down provides a general idea of how toxic that fat consumed was. Very unhealthy fats combined with an abnormal insulin receptor can lead to persistently elevated blood glucose levels for even days.

At least initially, the 3-hour post-meal glucose test should be done with every meal. From a practical point of view, this means the person should not be planning on going to bed for at least four hours, just in case the 3-hour glucose is higher than the 2-hour glucose. It should be done more than once for a specific meal, in order to confirm consistent results. Avoid mixing different fats during this phase. Ideally and to obtain more accurate results, a person could eat a larger than usual amount of the specific fat to be tested.

Although eating at restaurants is not recommended in the beginning, eventually this testing will allow deciding which restaurants and meals are safe to eat.

The easiest way to carry out this testing is with an implantable glucose monitoring device. The sensor needs to be replaced every several days depending on the model, usually ten to 14 days. Some have a low glucose alarm, a feature very useful when insulin resistance is improving, and diabetic medication dosage needs to be adjusted. Nevertheless, the old fashion finger stick is perfectly acceptable and probably a good option for those with prediabetes or those with diabetes who are still not taking any diabetic medications because insurance companies will not cover the implantable monitoring device.

2. MAXIMUM CHALLENGE 3-HOUR POST-MEAL HOME GLUCOSE TESTING.

This is the Cadillac diagnostic tool for discovering offending fats. In fact, this test is even more important for the fine tuning and reversal of insulin resistance. I struggled for some time until I implemented this testing. My fasting blood glucoses were still within normal limits but higher than expected. On first impression, I was not eating any unhealthy food products. The prior day 3-hours post-meal glucose tests were normal; thus, it did not seem any specific fats were negatively affecting my insulin receptor. These apparent contradictory findings lead me to the developing of the maximum challenge testing. This test allowed me to find which ones were the apparently benign fats or food products that were giving me mild but unexpected increase in my fasting blood glucose.

When the amount of fat consumed is small, a maximum challenge 3-hour post-meal home glucose testing is indicated. Another indication for this test is when it is not clear whether a specific fat is having a negative effect. As an example, one boiled egg might not cause insulin resistance, but this result does not completely rule out a negative effect on the insulin receptor. A better test for commonly eaten fats is to use the maximum challenge testing. In this case, a larger amount of fat should be consumed. For example, instead of eating one egg, consume four eggs or egg yolks. If this test still does not cause any insulin resistance, this fat cooked in that specific manner is safe at this time. Because higher temperatures will negatively affect fats, this test would need to be repeated if the fat ingested is the same but has been cooked at higher temperatures. Over time and when the insulin receptor improves, a specific fat might not give an abnormal test result any longer.

The maximum challenge test is useful to evaluate commercial food products that are usually consumed in small amounts. For example, expensive chocolate. Now you have the excuse to eat a much larger amount, all in the name of scientific evaluation. Unfortunately, if insulin resistance is detected, that specific food product should be avoided instead of just minimized. The goal is to avoid a cumulative or "repetitive like" injury.

SUMMARY OF CHAPTER

The combination of the 3-hour post meal glucose testing and the maximum challenge 3-hour post meal glucose testing is described. These testing will facilitate reversing insulin resistance. Both tests are needed to achieve good long-term glucose control.

CHAPTER 5. PROTOCOL FOR REVERSING DIABETES

5.1. PATIENTS WITH AN ELEVATED FASTING INSULIN LEVEL (most people).

This group includes most patients, certainly all patients with early disease. Treatment of diabetes should be based on avoiding foods that cause insulin resistance and life-style changes to improve insulin sensitivity.

Insulin resistance takes many years to develop, in most cases. Improving the insulin receptor is a slow process, it might take a few months. Blood glucose will improve faster but quickly reverting to old eating habits will cause an abnormally high blood glucose again. We are talking about life-style changes, a life-long term commitment. The rewards of following healthy habits will be great at the end. Minor setbacks during this process are expected and should not cause any anxiety because stress is a contributor to all chronic degenerative conditions.

Blood glucose needs to be controlled quite carefully while insulin resistance is being reversed. With improved insulin sensitivity, the need for diabetic medications will decrease or be eliminated. Patients on insulin must be extremely careful to avoid a dangerously low blood glucose. Continuous glucose monitoring devices are very useful because the alarm will sound if glucose drops to a certain level. In short, monitor blood glucose frequently and adjust medications accordingly.

CURE OR PREVENT DIABETES

5.1.1. INITIAL FAST (5-DAY FAST)

A 5-day fast is the ideal way to start although not mandatory. The traditional water fast is difficult for many people to follow, thus, not my recommendation even though it has been medically proven to be safe.[1] The average fast time was seven days.[1] Nevertheless, if you can do it, please feel free to proceed. Daily healthy salt should be included, could be in the form of broth. Healthy salts include Himalayan, Mediterranean, Celtic Sea, and Redmond salts. Some experts discourage exercising during a 5-day fast although there is no good scientific evidence against it. The sixth day should be a soft diet, this is not the time to celebrate and overeat.

Fasting will promote autophagy, a rejuvenating and self-cleaning process that might decrease cancer risk and is quite healthy. During autophagy cells will recycle old organelles. Stem cells will be released into the circulation after 3 days of fasting, this is the reason to continue fasting for two more days, so that the stem cells can establish themselves. Whether those stem cells one day could cure type 1 insulin-dependent diabetes is not known.

A 5-day fast can be done as often as once a month, for patients with significant comorbidities or medical problems. Healthy young patients (> 35 years old) could fast once a year. The frequency could be increased to speed up the recovery of the insulin receptor but no more often than once a month.

A much more attractive and easy way to implement a 5-day fast is by eating less than 400 calories/day of a plant-based diet (mostly vegetables), low in fat, with no animal products. Protein should be minimized or completely avoided because it interferes with autophagy. Healthy salt should be added as needed. It should not be table salt but a healthy option, like one of the salts mentioned above. Vegetables can be prepared with a fat-free salad dressing described below. A small amount of oil can be added but be careful because calories will increase rapidly. I mostly eat raw or steamed vegetables, including spinach, kale, lettuce, carrots, cabbage, sauerkraut, etc., as well as a few steamed mushrooms. Also, miracle rice or noodles (Shirataki Konjac), which does not have calories but be careful because it can cause excess flatulence depending on the amount consumed.

Contraindications to a 5-day fast include children, pregnancy, malnourishment, and abnormal low weight or BMI (body mass index). Dr. Valter Longo has done studies with a fast-mimicking diet up to age 65. For older people, a consultation with an expert or a primary care physician would be in order.

5.1.2. INITIAL DIET AFTER THE 5-DAY FAST.

Due to the extensive use of unhealthy fats by the food industry, processed foods should be completely avoided, at least until glucose has normalized. Later, the 3-hour post-meal glucose testing could be used to determine their effect on the insulin receptor but still minimizing processed food if not completely avoiding them. I personally do not eat any processed foods.

The initial diet should be a raw plant-based diet, at least for one month. Steamed vegetables are healthy and should be part of this diet, including broccoli, kale, Brussel sprouts, spinach, etc.

CURE OR PREVENT DIABETES

Patients with diabetic neuropathy (nerve pain) might need to remain on a plant-based diet. In this case, essential amino acids might need to be added to the diet to prevent deficiencies.

Although calorie counting is not needed, the insulin receptor will recover faster on a low-calorie diet. This is easily achieved when eating a low-fat plant-based diet. The body needs healthy fats for proper function but for the initial diet is better to stay on a low-fat diet, about 10% of calories from fat. This allows the body to start using the fat located inside the cell membranes. Once insulin sensitivity has been restored, the amount of fat can be slowly increased with careful monitoring of blood glucose levels.

Several medical articles have found better glucose levels when three meals, including breakfast, are consumed instead of the usual two meals during restricted feedings. But other studies have shown just the opposite, one concluding that eating two larger meals a day was better. To initially normalize blood glucose, I favor restricted feedings. Some people will call this "intermittent fasting" but this terminology is incorrect because fasting requires at least 24 hours without food intake. Restricted feeding implies eating all meals in a 4 to 6-hour time frame. It will give a person a better chance to quickly achieve a normal blood glucose so that the 3-hour glucose testing can be implemented. The 3-hour post-meal testing should be started as soon as blood glucose levels have normalized. If blood glucose does not normalize, then the 3-hour post-meal testing could be done to rule out offending fats. Once insulin sensitivity is normal, eating two versus three meals a day should not make a difference.

Avoiding a high-fat diet seems to be a good idea, at least initially. Even when glycemia (blood glucose) has normalized, it is prudent to avoid excess fat intake to decrease the risk of developing recurrent insulin resistance. Nevertheless, it might be possible to eat a large amount of certain healthy unheated fats without any negative consequences. This is something every individual will have to figure-out on his or her own.

Avoid eating at restaurants. Fast food should always be avoided, no exceptions to this rule. Fast food restaurants cook with processed vegetable oils, often reusing them, and this will harm the insulin receptor.

5.1.3. FOLLOW UP DIET.

Eventually, cooking is allowed. At least initially, start cooking at the lowest temperature possible and ideally without oil. Oil can be added later, something it was done a hundred years ago. If fat is used for cooking, it would be reasonable to use the most heat-resistant fats like butter, lard, or coconut oil. Coconut oil would be ideal as it does not seem to cause insulin resistance.

My advice is to avoid processed food altogether, even if insulin sensitivity normalizes, because it is very unhealthy and proinflammatory. The same applies to refined carbohydrates (e.g., bread, pasta, grain flower, cereals, etc.) and all unhealthy fats.

Good cell function depends on having healthy cell membranes. Both omega 3 and omega 6 fatty acids are needed for this purpose. A deficiency in omega 3 will disrupts good cell function. The ideal omega 6:3 ratio is 1:1 and it should be no greater than 3:1. Plant-based omega 3 fatty oils are not easily converted to the fatty acids the cells need. For this reason, it is advisable to take supplements of high-quality fish oil. One teaspoon (5 ml) daily, up to 3 teaspoons daily (15 ml). Make sure the manufacturer does routine mercury testing. It should be fish oil of known origin, not the more inexpensive capsules of unknown origin. The oil in those capsules might have been processed at temperatures higher than ideal. In some studies, taking fish oil capsules worsened outcomes. Another option is to take the same amount of cod liver oil, which has less omega 3 fatty acids but more vitamin A, which is needed for good immune function. Excess vitamin A becomes quickly toxic, thus avoid vitamin A supplements if you are already ingesting cod liver oil.

Even if insulin resistance subsides, food should never be cooked at high temperatures because it creates unhealthy byproducts, like carcinogens (cancer producing chemicals).

Which diet is healthiest is controversial, at least for those people with diabetes. In a study that included 129,716 patients followed for 26 years, the lowest all-cause and lowest cardiovascular disease mortality was found in the vegetable-based low-carbohydrate diet.[2] Eating a large amount of non-root vegetables (over the ground vegetables), like kale, spinach, broccoli, cauliflower, cabbage, etc., seems to be the best option.

My advice is to remain on an organic plant-based diet supplemented with a small amount of fat-free animal protein, at least for some time. Why? Because even a small amount of animal products increases the risk of diabetes. Chiu et al. [3] found that even a very small amount of animal products was detrimental, and no cases of diabetes were found among vegans. Just eating meat once a week (or more often) increases the risk of developing diabetes even after controlling for weight.[4] Eventually and with time, many people will be able to eat again animal fat that has not been overheated if the 3-hour post meal glucose test remains normal.

Unfortunately, vegans can suffer nutritional deficiencies and must take vitamin B12 supplements to prevent complications. Consuming all essential amino acids while on a vegan diet would take sophisticated knowledge and time. The solution to this problem is simple. A plant-based diet can be supplemented with fat-free animal protein. Daily supplementation with the 9 essential amino acids will solve this issue and this supplement is commercially available. Less expensive is to take whey protein isolate from grass fed cows, obviously in a larger amount since only about half of whey are essential amino acids. A more appealing way for others might be eating boiled egg whites without the yolks. Choose free-range eggs if you can.

What constitutes the ideal diet is confusing because not every diet is best for a specific person, condition, or age group. In addition, some scientific information seems to be contradictory. A widespread wrong notion is that high-protein diets are healthy. High-protein animal diets are very unhealthy, they increase chronic degenerative conditions and cancer. A large amount of protein might be beneficial for children and teenagers when they are developing muscle mass. Later in life, though, excess protein triggers the mTOR gene or pathway, increasing cancers among many other diseases. Too much animal protein is acidic, something that favors the growth and multiplication of viral infections, cancers, and nanobots. Better longevity has been achieved on a low-protein diet in adults under age 65.[5] One could reasonably question, how can a diabetes reversal diet be low-protein and relatively low-fat when a low carbohydrate diet offers better longevity? There are certainly no restrictions on how much healthy fat a person without insulin resistance may eat. As total fat can be a contributing factor to diabetes, the best diet will include a large amount of over-the-ground vegetables. Oils should be consumed in moderation. Many salads and dishes benefit from a fat-free dressing to minimize how much oil or fat is used. A simple and delicious fat-free dressing consists of same amounts of organic coconut aminos and organic apple cider vinegar. Liquid stevia or monk fruit may be added to taste.

Do not eat at fast food restaurants, even if your diabetes normalizes. It might be possible to make an occasional exception going to good restaurants and selecting your food choices very carefully. This will take some research and glucose testing.

Several studies have failed to find a correlation between protein and insulin resistance. Although animal products cause insulin resistance, fat is the culprit not protein. Some authors thought, at least in the past, that "high-quality" protein (usually animal in origin) helped diabetes. Unfortunately, there is no evidence to claim protein improves insulin sensitivity. How can it be that many patients feel animal products improve their blood glucose? The answer is obvious. Animal protein is a potent stimulator of insulin secretion. Thus, after eating animal protein there will be more circulating insulin in the blood, which will decrease blood glucose levels. This sounds good to keep stable blood glucose levels. In fact, prestigious physicians have recommended many meals per day (like at least 6), with "high-quality" protein with every meal. Long-term, though, this is a recipe for disaster for several reasons. First, insulin is needed for survival, but high chronic levels are quite harmful because insulin is proinflammatory. In other words, high insulin levels lead to chronic inflammation which is the main cause of modern chronic degenerative diseases, like heart disease, heart attacks, stroke, high blood pressure, obesity, etc. Second, high insulin levels lead to obesity because insulin locks fat in the adipose tissue, not allowing the body to use body fat for energy. By gaining weight, insulin resistance worsens thus leading to higher insulin levels, a bad vicious cycle. This can become a spiraling down disaster, difficult to stop. Third, increasing the amount of animal products consumed also increases the amount of toxins ingested. It is estimated that 90% of toxins ingested are from animal products, only 10% from plant-based foods. Many of those toxins produce or worsen diabetes (see part 3 of this book for a detailed explanation). To decrease the toxic load, always eat ORGANIC food.

No specific changes need to be made for protein intake. It is possible that in a non-polluted planet, free of processed and unhealthy foods, that excess animal protein might not be harmful, but this is not the case in our modern Western societies.

While still in insulin resistance, carbohydrates should be minimized. Later, with time, there will be no restrictions. Nevertheless, refined carbohydrates should never become part of a healthy diet. How well diabetes is controlled can be determined with serial A1c hemoglobin, like every three months. One way to improve your A1c is to exercise after eating, if carbohydrates were a significant part of the meal. For example, walking fast one thousand steps at one, two, and three hours after the end of the meal will lower the post meal glucose curve. Abstaining from carbohydrates 3 hours before bedtime is also advisable. In general, not eating 2-3 hours before going to bed is healthy. If you cannot avoid snaking before going to bed, eat foods without carbohydrates, like fat bombs, olives, an avocado, or something similar. Carbohydrate intake just before bedtime will increase blood glucose, which will stay elevated for many hours because no significant physical activity takes place during sleep.

Comments on diabetic neuropathy. It is a debilitating painful condition, not curable with diabetic medications. Treatment with other medications, like Lyrica or gabapentin, is only symptomatic and does not slow down the progression of this condition. Fortunately, most diabetic patients do respond to a 100% plant-based diet. Usually, pain will subside within a few days. Actual nerve damage will take many months to normalize. 90% of toxins ingested with food come with animal products. Why neuropathy (pain) symptoms improve so much and so fast on a plant-based diet is not well understood but it might be due to the much lower toxin load of a plant-based diet compared to a mostly animal diet. If this is correct, it further supports the role of detoxification for diabetes.

5.1.4. MAXIMUM CHALLENGE 3-HOUR POST-MEAL HOME GLUCOSE TESTING.

Ideally, every fat consumed should be tested with the maximum challenge 3-hour post-meal glucose testing. This will take quite a bit of time and effort but some of the results will be surprising and unexpected. Innocuous appearing meals or fats will be found to be harmful. Whether a mildly offending fat can be eating or should be avoided is questionable. It should not be eaten initially for sure. Maybe in moderation later if insulin resistance does not recur on the 3-hour post-meal glucose testing and A1c remain stable and within normal limits. I personally stay away from any mildly offending fats.

This test is even more important with processed foods, if any are consumed, because it is not possible to know for sure how the ingredients were processed or whether interesterified fats are included. Of course, the best approach is eliminating processed foods all together. If a small amount of processed food is going to be introduced in the diet, they must be tested with the maximum challenge 3-hour post meal glucose testing.

5.1.5. NUTRITIONAL MODIFICATIONS & CHANGES MADE BASED ON THE 3-HOUR POST-MEAL HOME GLUCOSE TESTING.

Once an offending fat has been identified, it should be eliminated from the diet because the insulin receptor cannot be "cured" with current technology (although part 3 discusses a non-official approach on how to "cure" the insulin receptor). This is of critical importance. If hidden foods are causing insulin resistance, they must be identified and eliminated for long term success.

After a while, the 3-hour test might normalize with a specific meal that caused insulin resistance in the past. Although is very tempting to resume eating this food product, do not do so routinely.

5.1.6. CORRECT MINERAL DEFICIENCIES

CURE OR PREVENT DIABETES

Start with a hair tissue mineral analysis (HTMA) test. Unfortunately, usually it is not covered by insurance companies because official medicine has not caught up with this knowledge. Modern official medicine is focusing on treatment not on prevention. Functional (integrative) physicians have been aware of the usefulness of a hair tissue mineral analysis test for a long time. Blood test can easily miss deficiencies of intracellular minerals, like magnesium and potassium.

Any mineral deficiencies should be corrected accordingly. Of course, mineral supplementation will not improve insulin sensitivity if no mineral deficiency exists.

Chromium deficiency is the best known in diabetes and must be corrected. Like other minerals, chromium supplements will not improve insulin sensitivity in somebody who does not have a chromium deficiency. The best option is chromium polynicotinate. For example, ChromeMate® 200 mcg to 600 mcg daily.

Magnesium supplements should be considered by everybody because about 80-90% of our population has a magnesium deficiency. Magnesium is needed for more than 250 enzymatic reactions and it is necessary for energy production. A reasonable supplement dose is 400 mg to 1,000 mg of magnesium daily. It might need to be taken it in divided doses if it causes any diarrhea or gastrointestinal symptoms. Magnesium oxide should be avoided because its absorption rate is only 8%. A good compromise for effectiveness/price is magnesium citrate, which can be purchased bulk in powder form. More bio available magnesium varieties can be purchased but are more expensive.

Deficiencies in vanadium and copper should be corrected, also. All these minerals are available as nutritional supplements.

A commercially available product which includes mineral and other supplements is Carlson's product *Nutra-Support Diabetes* **https://www.carlsonlabs.com/nutra-support-diabetes.html**

5.1.7. EXERCISE

Exercise has been known to help insulin sensitivity for a very long time. Sedentary lifestyles increase insulin resistance by decreasing the number of mitochondria in muscles cells and because lack of exercise is a contributor to obesity (official accepted knowledge by conventional Medicine).

Well-designed exercise if the most effective way to increases the number of mitochondria in muscle cells, which will greatly increase insulin sensitivity. Mitochondria are the energy factories in the cells. Nothing can survive or remain healthy without appropriate energy production. Many over-the-counter supplements have been used to increase energy production at the cellular level. But the most effective and inexpensive way is with physical activity. In addition, exercise helps eliminating body toxins.

Not all types of exercise are the same or as effective for improving insulin sensitivity. Traditionally and for many decades, aerobic exercise was promoted. For example, running on a treadmill for one hour, four or five days per week. Long term, most people did not continue this type of activity. Although aerobic exercise is better than no exercise at all, today other forms of physical activity have been proven to be much more effective and practical. In general, exercise against resistance is better than aerobic activities.

What is the ideal exercise to increase the number of mitochondria? Considering the time-effort/new mitochondria ratio, an ideal exercise is high intensity interval training (HIIT) because it only needs to be done for 15-20 minutes, three or four times weekly. Many scientific studies have proven HIIT is significantly better then aerobic exercise. The increase in growth hormone and mitochondrial numbers are superior. It should be done at least twice a week. I personally do HIIT on a stationary bicycle in the basement of my house, which saves me time compared to going to a gymnasium.

Another attractive exercise is slow motion strength training. It has a big advantage, only needs to be done for 30 minutes once a week. A good book to get started with this type of exercise is *THE SLOW BURN FITNESS REVOLUTION* from Frederick Hahn, Michael R. Eades, M.D., and Mary Dean Eades, M.D. No good studies have compared this exercise to HIIT for improving insulin resistance. Personally, I favor HIIT or a combination of HIIT with slow motion exercise. Much more information is available for HIIT than slow motion exercise.

5.1.8. WEIGHT CONTROL

Losing weight and keeping the weight off can be a challenging endeavor. First, start with a plant-based ketogenic diet with a large amount of leafy vegetables, for at least one month. No animal products or alcohol are allowed initially. If it fails, metabolic disorders like low thyroid function might need to be ruled out. Persistent obesity could also be due to insulin resistance with high insulin levels, this can become a vicious cycle difficult to break. You may consider some diets like the plan Z diet or the HCG diet. The latter works better if the injections are used instead of oral HCG. An animal protein ketogenic diet might decrease weight significantly but has many long-term side effects and should not be continued for too long (a few months only).

When weight is lost, toxins that had accumulated in the fatty tissue are released. This is very unhealthy, and some patients will have significant symptoms, like anxiety, feeling poorly, etc. Thus, persons losing weight should always include some type of detoxification protocol. See chapter 7 for practical advice.

Interestingly, improving insulin sensitivity will help weight loss. Losing weight becomes very difficult, if not impossible, when circulating insulin levels are abnormally high. Insulin "locks" fat in the adipose tissue, not allowing the body to use it as an energy source.

Like with any other chronic conditions, the best approach to obesity is prevention which is difficult when people are bombarded with all types of toxins and processed foods.

5.1.9. STRESS CONTROL

Chronic stress is very harmful, not just for diabetes but many other conditions like heart disease. It increases cortisol levels, a hormone that increases insulin resistance and fat deposits. Cortisol also depresses the immune system. Stress should be avoided as much as possible. The best way to decrease chronic stress is with meditation. Five to fifteen minutes of daily meditation will suffice. Deep breathing exercises are good but in one study they did not decrease inflammatory markers as much as meditation.

5.1.10. CIRCADIAN RHYTHMS

Respect your circadian rhythms because the human body depends on them for good health. All body cells follow a circadian rhythm. Sleep about 8 hours a day, always at the same time if possible. Sleep deprivation is quite harmful in the long run. It negatively affects the immune system, insulin sensitivity, increases blood pressure, worsens concentration, and the list goes on and on.

Exposure to bright lights at night is not advisable. Amber glasses can be worn 2-3 hours before going to bed to block blue light, which interferes with the production of melatonin, a hormone needed for good sleep and health. All computer and television screens, cell phones, tablets, etc., produce a significant amount of blue light. Exposure to LED light is probably not healthy and certainly will not be good to produce melatonin at night.

5.1.11. DETOXIFICATION, DETOXIFICATION, DETOXIFICATION.

Detoxification is discussed in chapter 7 of the book. Detoxification is very important and deserves its own subchapter. "Detoxification, detoxification, detoxification" refers to the wide variety of toxins that potentially can negatively affect the insulin receptor. Often, it is a synergistic effect of several toxins combined what damages the insulin receptor.

5.1.12. SUPPLEMENTS

Supplements alone will not be effective if a person continuous eating unhealthy fat. It seems reasonable to take supplements initially until good glucose control has been achieved but do not expect any miraculous improvement with supplements alone. They should be used in conjunction with other remedies and making sure offending contributors are avoided. Once insulin resistance has normalized, you may decrease or stop taking supplements as tolerated.

There is a long list of supplements that have been found to improve insulin resistance. Unfortunately, it is not known which combination of supplements works best. Often 80% of the benefit comes from just 20% of the supplements taken.

It makes sense taking vitamin D3, 4,000-5,000 IU daily, because it has many other health benefits. Polyphenols found in cocoa, green tea, and apples are beneficial. Also, hibiscus tea, which helps heart disease.

Other beneficial supplements include:

Cinnamon ½ teaspoon daily. It can be sprinkled in other foods or placed in a smoothie. It should be organic Ceylon cinnamon because it has a much lower coumarin level.

Resveratrol 1,000 mg daily. It increases energy production.

CURE OR PREVENT DIABETES

Ginger 3 grams daily or three 1 gram capsules of ginger powder.

Cumin 2 grams daily.

Gymnema sylvestre 500-1,000 mg daily or 250 mg twice daily.

Milk thistle extract 1,000 mg daily.

African Mango 5,000 mg daily.

Trans-ferulic acid 500 mg daily.

Bitter melon 600 mg daily or 50-100 ml of juice daily).

Fish oil (1-2 grams daily). It must be high quality fish oil of known origin not fish oil capsules that might have mercury and might have been exposed to high heat during processing.

DHEA 100 mg daily.

Alpha lipoic acid 600-1,000 mg daily.

Beta glucans 500 mg daily.

You may also consider:

Turmeric (250 mg of curcumin daily).

Olive leaf extract.

Black seed 2 g/day.

Spirulina 2-3 g/day, although up to 19 g/day have been used:
https://www.ncbi.nlm.nih.gov/pubmed/12639401 and
https://www.ncbi.nlm.nih.gov/pubmed/30532573

Ginseng 1-3 g/day.

Berberine, 900-1,200 mg daily, although this supplement is more controversial.

Alpha-Cyclodextrin 2,000 mg before meals three times daily has been used both to lose weight and improve blood sugars.

5.1.13. WHAT TO DO WHEN THE OFFENDING FOOD DOES NOT CAUSE 3-HOUR INSULIN RESISTANCE ANY LONGER.

Eventually, the insulin receptor may normalize. This can take many months or even years. How do you know when the insulin receptor is working well? Repeat an offending meal (fat) in the same amount it used to cause insulin resistance in the past. At this time, the 3-hour glucose level will be lower than the 2-hours level and should be within normal limits. The question at this time is whether a person could start eating that specific fat or that fat cooked at that specific temperature. The answer to this question is not known but unhealthy fats (like trans fats, processed vegetable oils, and interesterified fats) should never be consumed. If you decide to eat that meal or fat, do it prudently, minimizing how much you consume and occasionally check a 3-hour post-meal glucose and follow your A1c. If enough unhealthy fats are consumed, insulin resistance will recur.

5.1.14. ALTERNATIVE TREATMENT (NON-TRADITIONAL): CDS

Discussion of CDS (chlorine dioxide solution) is under DETOXIFICATION PROTOCOLS in chapter 7.

5.2. PATIENTS WITH LOW FASTING INSULIN LEVEL.

A small percentage of diabetic patients will have chronic pancreatic beta cell damage. This will cause a lower insulin production than expected. Chronic inflammation finally took its toll on beta pancreatic cells, which inevitably succumb to the on slaughter. At this stage, reversing diabetes is much more difficult if possible.

5.2.1. FIVE DAY FAST.

It might be possible to regenerate new beta pancreatic cells by doing a 5-day fasting or a 5-day fast mimicking diet. This approach was proposed by a world-known researcher specializing in longevity, Valter Longo, Ph.D. Dr. Longo has done extensive studies and he concludes a 5-day fast mimicking diet is as good as the old fashion 5-day water fast. A 5-day fast mimicking diet is plant-based totaling about 800 calories per day. You may Google fast mimicking diets. A commercially available 5-day fast mimicking diet is also available (https://prolonfmd.com/); proceeds are used to continue research in this area.

The mechanism is simple. Fasting or fast mimicking diet will allow new stem cells to enter the circulation after three days of fasting. During the last two days of the five-day fast, stem cells will multiply and create new cells where needed. Whether this approach one day could cure or benefit type 1 insulin dependent diabetes is not known.

 How often a 5-day fast should be done is not known for sure, but it would be reasonable to do a 5-day fast once a month for at least one year, then tailor the frequency as appropriate.

5.2.2. OTHER INTERVENTIONS

Other interventions are the same as described for patients with a high fasting insulin level.

SUMMARY OF CHAPTER

Most patients will fit in the category of an elevated insulin level and this is good news. The 3-hour post meal glucose testing and the maximum challenge 3-hour post meal glucose testing will be used to find out and eliminate harmful fats and meals. An initial 5-day fast is recommended but not mandatory. The follow up diet will be mostly organic plant-based, eliminating processed foods, refined carbohydrates, and all unhealthy fats. Mineral deficiencies must be corrected.

CURE OR PREVENT DIABETES

Other helpful measures will be physical exercise (ideally HIIT), weight control, meditation for chronic stress control, respect circadian rhythms, detoxify toxins, and a combination of supplements. Patients with pancreatic cell damage and low insulin levels may not improve but should try 5-day fasting or 5-day fast mimicking diet.

B. CURING DIABETES (HEALING THE INSULIN RECEPTOR)

CHAPTER 6. ETIOLOGY (WHAT HARMS THE INSULIN RECEPTOR).

Based on the rapid increased of worldwide diabetes, it seems clear other factors causing diabetes are not understood or acknowledge by conventional Medicine.

To the possible surprise of the reader, environmental and food toxins are the main cause of diabetes. How can this be? Earlier in the book fats were to blame. It seems to be a clear contradiction, but the explanation is quite simple. Offending fats do not cause insulin resistance when the insulin receptor is normal. Those fats did not cause insulin resistance to the same person years earlier and they do not cause insulin resistance in people with a healthy insulin receptor. This is the reason why only avoiding offending fats will reverse diabetes but will not cure it, because it does not resolve the underlying metabolic problem which is a defective or harmed insulin receptor. Toxins damage the insulin receptor, thus becoming the initial or original cause of insulin resistance. Toxins decrease energy production at the level of the mitochondria, which leads to insulin resistance. Once the insulin receptor is malfunctioning, unhealthy fats or heated healthy fats build up inside the cell (as lipid deposits), finally blocking the receptor. This will abnormally increase blood glucose levels. Toxins are the original culprit; fats are the secondary and more visible cause. An elevated blood glucose is the messenger, thus, "do not shoot the messenger", which happens to be the carbohydrates in this case. Unhealthy fats, though, are toxic and should be added to the list of toxins harming the insulin receptor. This fact seems to confuse some people. Processed GMO (genetically modified) vegetable oils come with significant number of toxins, acquired while the plants were growing and were spread with chemical fertilizers and pesticides. In addition, more toxins are added later during industrial processing. All man-made fats harm the insulin receptor.

Toxins causing diabetes are called "diabetogens." Many diabetogens also cause obesity. Thus, obesity and diabetes correlate quite well. Conventional Medicine thinks obesity causes diabetes, but correlation does not prove causation. It certainly could be that the same toxins causing obesity are causing diabetes. A study from Lee et al.[1] stated that "obesity did not increase the prevalence of diabetes among subjects with nondetectable levels of POPs (persistent organic pollutants) even though there were sufficient numbers of study subjects at risk in each BMI (body mass index) category." This article was based on the results from the National Health and Examination Survey 1999-2002. The study also found that persons with the highest blood levels of POPs had about 38 times higher risk to develop diabetes than those people with the lowest levels. How much is 38 times more? Twice more is a 100% increase. Thus, 38 times more is a 3,800% increase. Can you imagine if you could increase your financial investment by 3,800%? Age was the factor that strongest correlated with the amount of POPs found in people.[1] This is the price to pay for living in a polluted planet. From a diabetes treatment point of view, it is important to know that 90% of the POPs come from animal foods consumed by the general population that does not have occupational or accidental exposures. This is a clear indication for diabetic patients to mostly switch to an organic plant-based diet.

CURE OR PREVENT DIABETES

Synthetic organic chemical production has increased drastically over the last few decades and this increase correlates quite well with diabetes prevalence.[2] About 80,000 chemicals are used at this time. The chemical industry does not have to prove chemicals are safe to humans or animals.

Considering current evidence, I am pretty sure all modern chronic degenerative conditions, including cancer, autoimmune diseases, heart disease, etc., are caused by a toxin overload and nutritional deficiencies.

There is a long list diabetogens. Most diabetogens decrease insulin sensitivity. Some include:

Dioxins used in a variety of industrial processes. Dioxins are considered POPs. Other POPs include chlordane, DDT, aldrin, endrin, dichlorodiphenyl, heptachlor, mirex, hexachlorobenzene, toxaphrene, furans, and PCBS. POPs are used in many industrial and manufacturing processes as well as in agriculture and disease control.

Bisphenol A (BPA), which is used to manufacture some plastics. Unfortunately, it is frequently used for plastics used for food storage. It is also used for drinking bottles and in the liner of food cans. BPA is a very harmful endocrine disrupter, contributing to many other health problems like breast and prostate cancers, and heart disease.

Phthalates are used in plastics to extend their durability and flexibility as well as in many cosmetic and other products used by humans.

Organochlorine pesticides, which farmers use in absurd amounts. Pesticides also contaminate the air around farms and drinking water. Glyphosate, an herbicide, is the main ingredient in RoundUp.® Much better studied is agent orange, which causes multiple medical diseases, including an increased risk of diabetes. Both products are similar.

Polycyclic aromatic hydrocarbons considered to be the main carcinogen in tobacco smoke.

Heavy metals. Arsenic is an exception and instead of decreasing insulin sensitivity it harms pancreatic cells decreasing insulin production. It contaminates foods (like rice, poultry, and seafood) and drinking water. Other heavy metals include lead, cadmium, and mercury. All heavy metals are toxic to the human body. Many people group aluminum with heavy metals. Aluminum is the main cause of autism and many neurological diseases. Unfortunately, aluminum is frequently present in vaccines (after pharmaceutical companies were pressured to stop using mercury).

<u>SUMMARY OF CHAPTER</u>

Most modern chronic medical conditions, including diabetes, heart disease, strokes, obesity, high blood pressure, cancer, autoimmune diseases, arthritis, osteoarthritis, osteoporosis, dementia, autism and other neurological conditions, depression, etc., are caused by toxins and nutritional deficiencies. Once toxic load exceeds the capacity of the human body to detoxify itself, diseases start happening. Diabetes is not an exception. Multiple toxins are responsible for damaging the insulin receptor, causing insulin resistance (thus, diabetes).

CHAPTER 7. CURING THE INSULIN RECEPTOR: DETOXIFICATION PROTOCOLS.

Something wonderful about these detoxification protocols is that they can be used to prevent or improve the great majority of chronic medical conditions, including heart disease, high blood pressure, dementia, degenerative neurological diseases, and so on.

Although not used by most conventional physicians, it is a good idea to do a hair tissue mineral analysis (HTMA) test. This test provides good evidence of chronic toxin load in the body. Specific therapies can be directed to eliminate the harmful toxins, but those details are beyond the scope of this book. Detoxification in general and specifically heavy metal detoxification is a slow process that will take a long time, months or years. Detoxification is like running a marathon. It would advisable to repeat the HTMA test one year later, and then as needed based on those results.

Medical providers specializing in detoxification are available, although not frequently sought by most people. My advice is to get professional help for this detoxification process. This field of Medicine is somewhat confusing because specialists call themselves many different names. The most frequently names used include Functional Medicine, Integrative Medicine, Naturopathic Medicine, Holistic Medicine, Alternative Medicine, and the Veterans Administration System uses the name Whole Health.

No randomized clinical trials have been performed to determine the best detoxification protocol. In fact, no randomizes trials have been performed to find out how effectively diabetes can be cured with detoxification. Unfortunately, the financial interest of our current medical system is to treat chronic medical conditions, no to prevent or reverse them. This will eventually change in the future, hopefully soon.

7.1. DECREASE EXPOSURE TO TOXINS.

First and foremost, avoid toxins as much as possible. Our environment is full of toxic chemicals, including detergents, deodorants, furniture and clothing with flame retardants, cosmetics, and a long list of other chemicals, too long to be included here. Disinfectants like DCP (dichlorophenol) increase the risk of diabetes.

Avoid all GMO foods, thus processed foods should not be purchased. Food should always be organic to decrease the pesticide load and because it has better nutritional value. Many GMO foods come with the herbicide glyphosate, considered a carcinogen by WHO (World Health Organization). Pesticides should be avoided. It is tempting to call the exterminator to spray your house for insects and mosquitoes, but do not. Permethrin, used for mosquito control, is unhealthy. Use safe mosquito repellants. If you still want to use deet, only use it on clothing that is not touching your skin.

Anytime you buy a product, check the Environmental Working Group's web page https://www.ewg.org/ to make sure your purchase is safe. An app can be downloaded into your smart phone so that you can scan commercially available products. Regarding skin products, do not use them unless you are willing to eat the ingredients because products placed on the skin are absorbed. For example, using almond or avocado oil for a skin massage is acceptable.

Avoid plastic containers. Use glass containers and bottles. Cookware should be stainless steel metal or have a ceramic coating. Teflon coated is harmful. Food should not get in contact with plastics. Also avoid drinks in aluminum containers.

Use a reverse osmosis system for all your cooking and drinking water. Fluoride found in city water has many adverse effects, including an increased risk of developing diabetes.

Get fresh air into your house and use an air filter to clean the air. Change air filters often.

Avoid heavy metals like copper cookware. Avoid anything that has aluminum, like cookware, some vaccines, and commercial baking powder. Do not drink from aluminum cans. Deodorants with aluminum increase the risk of breast cancer. Stop eating mercury. This will exclude big fish, like tuna. Avoid fish oil capsules and fish oil in general unless the manufacturer routinely tests for mercury.

Avoid fast food restaurants because the food is cooked with unhealthy oils, which often are reused.

Avoid as many chemicals as you can. If you can smell the chemical, it is getting into your body. You might like the smell of a new car, but you are breathing toxic fumes. The same applies to many other products, like new carpet and furniture, etc.

When you put gasoline in your car, do not breathe the fumes.

7.2. GENERAL DETOXIFICATION MEASURES.

Detoxification will not just help diabetes but many other medical conditions, like obesity, heart disease, and any other chronic inflammatory diseases.

Liver function. Although many organs detoxify the body, the main detoxifier is the liver, but it can only do so much. Interventions to improve liver function will help detoxification. Alcohol interferes with liver function, thus hindering the detoxification process. Detoxification by the liver requires proteins. During the acute detoxification process is probably not the best time to be on a low protein diet.

Weight loss. Losing weight will release toxins from the fatty tissue. Thus, some type of detoxification protocol should be implemented, including exercise which helps eliminating toxins.

Daily probiotics. I like better taking probiotics in the form of healthy food, like sauerkraut. Probiotic pills are expensive, but they are better than doing nothing.

CURE OR PREVENT DIABETES

Fiber intake. Increase fiber intake. The best way to do so is by switching to a mostly plant-based diet. Vegetable smoothies are a good way to get many nutrients and extra fiber. Freshly ground flax seeds are a good option.

Detoxifying foods. Increasing the amount of detoxifying foods is a good way to get started.

> Chlorella and spirulina, both 3 grams daily. Both can be ingested as food or be taken in a tablet form. Spirulina does not taste good and can ruin a smoothie. I take 3 grams of spirulina tablets daily.

> Chlorophyll. It is available in different preparations, I like the concentrated drops best, 50 mg under the tongue daily, up to three times a day.

> Cabbage and cabbage family vegetables.

> Cilantro, also available as a supplement. One teaspoon of cilantro leaves mixed with a smoothie daily.

> Cruciferous vegetables like broccoli, kale, and bok choy. Broccoli and kale should be steamed to prevent goiters.

> Onion, garlic both have sulfur-based components useful for detoxification.

> Ginger, turmeric.

> Parsley.

> Ground flax seeds.

> Brazil nuts or selenium supplements (about 50-60 mcg daily). Selenium is needed for detoxification. Just a few Brazil nuts daily usually provides the daily requirement but the amount per Brazil nut is quite variable. There is no need to take selenium supplements if you eat Brazil nuts.

> Coconut oil and ghee help detoxify fat soluble toxins. In fact, there is a one-week protocol eating ghee and avoiding any other fats (thus excluding meat and dairy) to eliminate persistent organic pollutants. Coconut oil also helps detoxify heavy metals.

The best way to eat a large amount of healthy vegetables is by drinking a vegetable smoothie daily or most days. My usual vegetable smoothie is 1-1.4 liters, 5-6 times a week.

Glyphosate is eliminated steadily by the body. Thus, the most important action you can take is to avoid GMO foods and exposure to RoundUp®. Cilantro, as a food or supplement, will help eliminate glyphosate.

Nutritional supplements.

> Glutathione should be liposomal or topical. If not, it is not very effective because it breaks down in the small bowel. A more practical and inexpensive approach is to take supplements of NAC, a precursor of glutathione. Glutathione is present in fresh fruits and vegetables, and even in larger amounts in sesame seeds.

NAC is N-acetyl L-cysteine and it is one of the most important supplements for detoxification. 600 mg twice daily.

DHA (100 mg/day), R lipoic acid (600 mg/day; doses have greatly varied in different studies, from 200 mg to 1,800 mg/day for 2 weeks to 1 year), PQQ (20 mg/day) may also be taken.

Milk thistle extract 4:1 500 mg (equivalent to 2,000 mg of milk thistle seed) before a meal daily.

Magnesium works both as a detoxifier and to increase energy production. 400 mg to 1,000 mg daily. Magnesium citrate is a good compromise for price/quality. It might need to be taken in divided doses to prevent diarrhea.

Vitamin B complex. Vitamin Bs increase energy production and are needed for many functions. Deficiencies in folic acid and other vitamin Bs should be corrected or you just may take a daily supplement. For example, folic acid 400 mcg daily, B_{12} 500 mcg of methyl cobalamin daily, B_2 10 mg daily, and B_5 250 mg daily.

Vitamin C 1,000 mg daily or twice daily. Ideal liposomal or extended release vitamin C.

Resveratrol increases the number of mitochondria, improving cellular energy production. 1,000 mg daily.

Molybdenum should be corrected. If deficient, take 200 mcg daily.

Zinc deficiency must be corrected. Take 25 mg daily if needed.

Calcium-D glucorate has also been used because it is converted into glucaric acid, which supports an important detoxification pathway in the liver. Glucoric acid is found in apples, oranges, cruciferous vegetables, and grapefruit. As a supplement, doses as high as 1,500-3,000 mg daily have been recommended.

Exercise. Exercise, like sweating, eliminates toxins. Any exercise is better than nothing, but HIIT (high intensity interval training) is advisable. Obviously, exercise should be tailored to the person's physical condition.

Massage therapy. Massages also help eliminating toxins. This is not the main detoxifying therapy, though.

Fasting. The health benefits of fasting are too numerous to enumerate. Fasting also helps the detoxification of the body. It can be done in many ways. As little as a 1-2 day fast will help. Some people will do "intermittent fasting" which is restricted feedings, eating all meals in a 4 to 8-hour period. The most effective way is the 5-day fast or fast mimicking diet. During this 5-day fast period other detoxifying measures can be continued, like exercise, sauna, and supplements like zeolite, bentonite clay, diatomaceous earth, and EDTA.

Hydration. Stay well hydrated since the kidneys excrete toxins. Switch from drinking water to organic hibiscus tea brewed at home using reverse osmosis filtered water. May alternate with organic green tea and matcha tea. Sweeten tea with organic liquid monk fruit or organic liquid stevia for taste. Hibiscus tea improves insulin sensitivity and decreases heart disease. Green and matcha tea are detoxifiers. Matcha tea has EGCG (epigallocatechin gallate), which has been shown to detoxify polychlorinated biphenyls. Tea will have more beneficial medical properties if is brewed using the correct method. Always pour boiling water directly on the tea. Do not follow the tea brewing instructions, which usually let the water cool down some after reaching boiling temperature. In addition, keep the tea in hot water for much longer then specified in the manufactures brewing instructions. The final tea might a bit stronger, even bitter, but it will be healthier. Monk fruit or stevia will take care of any possible bitterness.

Alkalinize the urine. More toxins will be reabsorbed when the urine is more acidic. To decrease urinary pH, eat a mostly plant-based diet with plenty of green leafy vegetables. For example, urine pH will decrease by eating stinging nettle (steamed, in a smoothie). Supplements to decrease urine's pH include sodium bicarbonate, potassium bicarbonate, magnesium citrate, and potassium citrate.

Supplements needed for general health. The following supplements are not specific detoxifiers but are essential for good health. The body needs them to function properly. Vitamin D3 5,000 IU daily, it should be taken with a meal to improve absorption. Vitamin D is not actually a vitamin but a hormone, which is needed for not just the bones but for the immune and arterial systems. Vitamin K2 is essential for good bone health, and to prevent ectopic calcifications and heart disease. It is available as MK4 and MK7. MK4 was used for several Japanese studies but needs to be taken at a higher dose and three times daily. In Western countries, MK7 is favored and can be taken only once a day, 100-300 mcg daily. It should be taken with a meal because it is liposoluble, thus it needs fat to be absorbed. Do not confuse vitamin K2 with K1, which is for clotting. Modern diets are not vitamin K1 deficient, thus you do not have to supplement it.

7.2. SAUNAS AND SAUNA PROTOCOL.

SAUNAS

Profuse sweating in saunas eliminates toxins, and this fact has been proven beyond reasonable doubt. Maybe this is the reason why there is an indirect correlation between the number of weekly saunas taken and the prevalence of heart disease (more saunas, less heart disease). Sauna therapy has been shown to improve cardiovascular disease, hypertension, congestive heart failure, anorexia nervosa, bipolar disorder, dementia, depression, chronic pain, autoimmune problems, and chronic fatigue. Saunas have a few contraindications, including aortic stenosis (narrowing), severe orthostatic hypotension (low blood pressure made worse when standing up), unstable angina (chest pain), and a recent heart attack. Some people will not advise saunas during pregnancy.

Sauna therapy eliminates multiple toxins, including heavy metals (mercury, lead, cadmium, nickel, and antimony), bisphenol A (BPA), phthalates, chlorinated pesticides, and polychlorinated biphenyls.

CURE OR PREVENT DIABETES

Saunas can be divided in traditional and infrared. Traditional saunas include radiant-heat and dry-heat, the difference is whether water is added to create steam. Traditional saunas are effective but in some studies they are not as good as infra-red saunas. How long to stay in the sauna is variable depending on many factors. From 15 to 60 minutes but get out if you feel uncomfortable. A steam sauna will be set at a lower temperature, 150-180 degrees Fahrenheit. A dry sauna needs a higher temperature to achieve the same amount of sweating. If the temperature is very high (> 200 degrees Fahrenheit), it might feel like the air is burning the nose. Most people prefer a steam sauna. Water steam is produced, traditionally, by pouring water on hot granite rocks. A more convenient way is using a sauna that has a steam unit. A combination of an actual steam unit and a sauna is quite a bit more expensive. More practical is to buy a sauna that has a water reservoir close to the heating, which will get the water to a boiling temperature. A good temperature in a wet sauna is between 160- and 180-degrees Fahrenheit, 15 to 30 minutes. Temperature and time in the sauna can be changed based on personal preference. I like being able to lay down, something I cannot do in the 1-2 person infrared sauna.

Infrared saunas are good for general detoxification. The traditional saunas are good but not as effective in eliminating body toxins, based on some studies although not everybody agrees on this point.

Infrared saunas penetrate deeper, are less expensive, use less energy, are portable, and can be plugged in to a 110-125 volt outlet. In other words, an infrared sauna can be mounted anywhere in the house. Many models for one or 1-2 persons are available online for home delivery. They have built in speakers; you can bring in your own MP3 music player. Another advantage of infrared saunas is they work well at a lower temperature. Usually 120-150 degrees Fahrenheit is enough, for 20-40 minutes depending on personal preference, up to one hour if you have that much time to spare. A one-person unit might be the best option, except for very large people. By being smaller, the infrared panels will be closer to the skin, increasing the beneficial effects. I set the temperature at the maximum possible, 151 degrees Fahrenheit in the case of my infrared sauna. The temperature usually will not get to 151 degrees, which means the unit stays on all the time, thus benefiting from continued infrared heat.

After using a sauna, water and electrolyte loses should be replaced accordingly. Electrolyte losses will be larger the first few times a sauna is used. Eventually, the body will adapt and lose less minerals.

SAUNA PROTOCOL

Several protocols have been described, including the Hubbard Method, the Rea Protocol, and the Crinnion Naturopathic Protocol.

The following is a simple-to-follow niacin, exercise, sauna protocol:

CURE OR PREVENT DIABETES

Take 100 mg of immediate release niacin. This dose can be increased as needed. Niacin will produce vasodilation (a skin flush) within 30-60 minutes. How much niacin to take is quite personal. I do not do well with 500 mg, I tend to get some nausea and dizziness, ending up leaving the sauna before my time was over. Niacin dose for flushing can be up to 1,000 mg per day. Chronic niacin intake can increase homocysteine levels in some patients, an independent factor for heart disease. Thus, do follow up blood testing to rule out increased homocysteinemia or take supplements consistent of folic acid (1 mg), vitamin B6 (5-20 mg), and vitamin B12 (400-1,000 mcg) daily.

Exercise right after taking niacin. The best exercise is HIIT. I use a stationary bike. If you prefer anaerobic exercise, you may do so up to one hour. One of many advantages of HIIT is that 15-20 minutes is enough.

Right after finishing exercising, get in the preheated sauna. My traditional sauna will be hot in about 10 minutes because uses about 8 KW of energy. I stop the HIIT exercise on the bike, turn the sauna on, and finish on the bike. My infrared sauna takes at least 15 minutes to heat well, thus I turn it on just before getting on the stationary bicycle. About 20-30 minutes in the sauna is enough time. You may weigh yourself before and after the sauna to get an idea how much are your fluid losses. It is nothing unusual to lose between ½ and 1 pounds, but you certainly may lose more.

Take a shower to wash off all toxins as soon as you finish the sauna. Make sure you replace fluid and electrolytes losses.

It is reasonable to take other detoxifying products around the sauna. Liposomal glutathione (350-500 mg) or NAC (600 mg) can be taken before and/or after the sauna (optional). Binding agents like bentonite clay, zeolite, diatomaceous earth, and activated charcoal can be taking to trap any toxins released into the gastrointestinal tract.

OTHER COMMENTS ON SAUNAS

How often should this protocol be used? In an acute therapy phase, 5-6 days/week is indicated. One you have reached the chronic state, once or twice every week is enough for maintenance.

What if you forget taking niacin? No problem, the protocol still works. What if you just do not have the time to exercise? No problem either. If you decide to skip the shower after the sauna, make sure you wipe off well all the sweat. The point I am trying to make is anything in the protocol can be skipped except for the sauna. It might take somewhat longer to obtain the same results, though.

7.3. ZEOLITE, CLAYS, DIATOMACEOUS EARTH.

ZEOLITE.

Zeolite is alkaline volcanic ash (clinoptilolite) that came in contact with the sea and it is an amazing detoxifier. It has a very high cation exchange capacity (CEC) of 120. This implies a great ability to remove heavy metals and other toxins from the body. It will stay in the body for 6-8 hours. It binds most tightly to mercury, then lead, tin, cadmium, arsenic, aluminum, antimony, iron, and nickel in descending order. More heavy metals can be detected in the urine within one week of taking zeolite. It also binds to other toxins like dioxins, pesticides, and PCPs.

Interestingly, zeolite also possesses other beneficial properties, including blocking viral replication, improving mood and liver function, and binding to mycotoxins (fungi, yeast). It provides other minerals, but this is only a minor secondary benefit. Zeolite has the potential to improve mineralization in the body, but this is probably due to the removal of heavy metals that are competing with essential metals.

Zeolite has no known side effects. It can be used in combination with other agents to maximize a detoxification protocol.

To be effective, zeolite must be micronized. A combination of small and larger particles is ideal. Although available in liquid form, choose powder zeolite.

Dose is 5 grams of powder (two teaspoons) diluted in water, three times daily for 90 days. Then decrease to 5 grams daily. Dose can be as high as 30-45 grams/day in divided doses.

BENTONITE CLAY.

Bentonite clay it also comes from volcanic ash trapped in an evaporated seabed. It is an absorbent aluminum phyllosilicate clay consisting mostly of montmorillonite.

It contains many minerals, including calcium, magnesium, silica, copper, iron, sodium, and potassium. Like zeolite, it has a negative charge which allows it to bind to heavy metals and other toxins, since most toxins are positively charged. Its CEC is very good, although not as high as zeolite, at about 80.

Bentonite clay come in two varieties, calcium bentonite and sodium bentonite. For detoxification, you should buy calcium bentonite. For those concerned with calcium supplements increasing the risk of heart disease, bentonite clay provides a rather small amount of calcium. Sodium bentonite is available in food grade, but it is mostly for industrial use.

Another option is Sacred Clay, a combination of several clays including bentonite clay.

Dose is 1-3 teaspoons dissolved in water daily. For metal detoxification the dose is one teaspoon three times daily. Maintenance dose is one teaspoon every 2-3 days. Some experts recommend hydrating bentonite clay in water for 6-18 hours, but others disagree and recommend drinking the mixture right away without waiting. I like the latter option.

To improve detoxification by bentonite clay, you may take cilantro 100 mg four times daily.

DIATOMACEOUS EARTH.

CURE OR PREVENT DIABETES

Diatomaceous Earth is diatoms, single celled life form. It has a negative charge and about 90% is silica, thus structurally is very small pieces of glass. This allows it to kill external insects as well as internal parasites, like worms, by literally cutting them. As a detoxifier, it attracts and bounds heavy metals, thus ideal for our purpose here. Although its CEC is much lower than zeolite, at 35-40, it still is very useful.

For human consumption and animal use diatomaceous earth should be food grade. Enter "FOOD CHEMICAL CODEX GRADE" in a search engine and you will find many products. I purchased a 50-pound bag since it has other applications. Non-food grade (pool grade) is calcined (treated with heat) and used in filters, thus, not appropriate for humans or animals.

Dosing. Start with one teaspoon dissolved in water daily, increasing to two teaspoons. Up to 1-2 tablespoons a day. It is taken on an empty stomach, at least one hour and two hours before and after meals, respectively.

RECOMMENDATION

All three products can be taking together to benefit from their synergistic effect. An intensive 3-month protocol followed by a maintenance dose and rechecking the hair analysis within one year seems reasonable. For the intensive protocol take Zeolite three times daily, bentonite clay and diatomaceous earth can be taken once or twice a day. Another option is to take all three of them twice daily. For maintenance, all three products can be taken once daily.

7.4. COMMENTS ON HEAVY METALS DETOXIFICATION.

COMMENTS ON EDTA

Heavy metals include lead, mercury, cadmium, sometimes chromium. Less commonly, other metals including iron, copper, zinc, aluminum, beryllium, cobalt, manganese, and arsenic may be considered heavy metals. From a detoxification point of view, we worry mostly about lead, mercury, cadmium, aluminum, and arsenic.

For heavy metals detoxification what works best is IV (intravenous) EDTA, an FDA approved therapy. EDTA is ethylenediaminetetraacetic acid. IV EDTA is expensive and should be done by a well-trained physician. A randomized trial should that IV EDTA decreased the risk of new heart attacks among diabetic patients. As a do it as a home remedy, another route must be considered.

Unfortunately, oral EDTA is very poorly absorbed by the gastrointestinal tract, only about 5%. EDTA suppositories are much better absorbed but this route is inconvenient and not practical for most people.

Of the non-liposomal oral EDTAs, the most cost-effective one is liquid EDTA. Cardio Renew® is a commercially available product (www.cardiorenew.com) that comes with good instruction for its use.

CURE OR PREVENT DIABETES

The most potent oral EDTA is the liquid liposomal form, albeit more expensive. Is it worth the extra cost? This might depend on the metal toxic load somebody suffers. It is certainly an attractive option for some patients. In addition, liposomal EDTA is available combined with R-Lipoic acid which has the advantage of crossing the brain blood barrier.

COMMENTS ON ALUMINUM DETOXIFICATION

Aluminum is very harmful to the brain and the body in general and it has become a major health problem due to the extensive use of aluminum for many purposes. Dr. Stephanie Seneff, senior MIT researcher, is convinced autism and many other neurological conditions are caused by the synergistic effect of aluminum combined with glyphosate.

Before you even think of detoxifying aluminum, you should first avoid any products with aluminum, like deodorants, baking soda, aluminum foil and cookware, and vaccines containing aluminum. Do not drink from aluminum cans.

Some aluminum is eliminated during a sauna, but this is not the preferred treatment modality.

A short-term therapy with horsetail will be beneficial. Horsetail is an herb; it can be consumed as a tea or as a supplement. The supplement can be purchased as a concentrated extract, which can be added to a smoothie. Long-terms consumption is not recommended because it can deplete other minerals. Horsetail works because it contains silica, which also can be found in diatomaceous earth.

The dose for food grade diatomaceous earth is one teaspoon in a glass of water daily. Over a few weeks, the dose can be increased to twice daily. Foods helping eliminating aluminum include garlic, parsley, cilantro, chlorella, spirulina, and organic coconut oil.

An alternative for diatomaceous earth is Zeolite.

DHA (precursor of several hormones, 100 mg daily), R lipoic acid (100 mg to 240 mg daily), and PQQ (increases the number of mitochondria, 20 mg daily) will help bring aluminum levels down.

Chlorella is also effective, take at least 3 grams daily.

Coconut oil has been used but should not be the main therapy.

7.5. ALTERNATIVE DETOXIFICATION PROTOCOL (NON-TRADITIONAL): CDS. THE MOST POWERFUL UNIVERSAL DETOXIFIER?

Could CDS be the holy grail of detoxification? An universal detoxifier? CDS is certainly not approved for human use by conventional Medicine. In fact, the FDA has stated it is dangerous and should not be consumed by human beings. But, are there any hidden financial interests trying to keep CDS off the public's radar? Several sources describe CDS but I like best Dr. Andreas Ludwig Kalcker. Dr. Kalcker has a Ph.D. in biophysics and has published a book on

CURE OR PREVENT DIABETES

CDS, which he has been researching for many years. Unfortunately, his book titled *FORBIDDEN HEALTH. INCURABLE WAS YESTERDAY* has been banned by the main book sellers in USA. This book still can be purchased from the publisher Voedia in Spain, at **https://voedia.com/en/** and Worldwide distributors can be found at https://voedia.com/en/content/7-distribuidores

CDS stands for chlorine dioxide solution. Chlorine dioxide is made by combining equal amounts of hydrochloric acid (4-5%) and sodium chlorite (25-28%) in a glass container. Dr. Kalcker uses 4% hydrochloric acid and 25% sodium chlorite but in USA it is easier to purchase 5% hydrochloric acid and 28% sodium chlorite (www.waterpureworld.com). Either combination is acceptable. Chlorine dioxide solution is when the gas produced by the reaction is stored in water. This is accomplished by keeping the mixed solution in a shot glass which is placed in a closed glass container for 12 hours, in a dark place at room temperature. This container must be cooled down before it is opened to get the chlorine dioxide solution (the water in the container) out of the glass container. This is done outside or in a well-ventilated area with an air suctioning system. CDS must be kept in the refrigerator because it evaporates at 52 degrees Fahrenheit. The reader must watch Dr. Kalcker videos to make CDS safely. CDS has a big advantage over chlorine dioxide because it is pH neutral. Chlorine dioxide mixed in water (not the gas in water) can be used instead of CDS, but its low pH can cause gastrointestinal symptoms, like diarrhea. Because it is not a gas, chlorine dioxide can be taken at room temperature. Finding Dr. Kalcker's videos might take some effort because YouTube takes them down. In my opinion, YouTube, Twitter, Facebook, Google, etc., take down or ban any information that goes against the big financial interests of the elites that currently control most of the world. Other people keep on uploading Dr. Kalckers' videos on YouTube but you might need to check others platforms like bitchute.com, d.tube, dailymotion, vimeo, or veoh.com. If everything fails, Dr. Kalcker's book describes the steps well. Dr. Kalcker has easy to follow instructions on this YouTube **https://www.youtube.com/watch?v=8CHEiLEJ_6k** that has been uploaded by somebody else after the original video was taken down. It might be banned already by the time you read this.

CDS is not bleach like some people with bad intentions have stated. How can CDS improve insulin resistance? The mechanism is not known for sure and it might be in several ways. CDS is an oxidizer which provides more oxygen to be used by mitochondria. Thus, CDS increases energy production in the mitochondria. Nothing works without energy. Cells need plenty of energy, if not enough is available the cells will not function properly. I think the main mechanism is probably as a detoxifier. This would explain why insulin resistance improves mostly after a few months and on a relatively higher dose of CDS, like 30 to 50 ml in a liter of water. The lowest dose for a CDS protocol is 10 ml of CDS in a liter of water, the maximum dose is 80 ml/L of water.

CDS is commercially available (www.waterpureworld.com) but not FDA approved for any medical conditions. It has been standardized to a 3,000 PPM (parts per million) solution. It is used in water purification. Making CDS at home is much more inexpensive and it is a very simple process but beyond the scope of this book.

CURE OR PREVENT DIABETES

<u>SUMMARY OF CHAPTER</u>

It is possible to cure diabetes by detoxifying the body. This will be a difficult and long process which will include:

-Decreasing exposure to toxins as much as possible.

-General detoxification measures.

-Implementing a sauna protocol.

-Implementing a Zeolite, Clays, and Diatomaceous Earth protocol.

-Detoxifying heavy metals with EDTA and other supplements.

-Consider taking the universal detoxifier CDS (chlorine dioxide solution).

C. AUTHOR'S PERSONAL EXPERIENCE

Quite a few years ago, while already on an organic diet, I decided to check my glyphosate levels (main ingredient in RoundUp^R) in the urine, assuming none would be detectable. To my surprise, a small amount of glyphosate was detected. This illustrates how difficult, if not impossible, is to stay away from harmful toxins despite making a very significant effort. Unfortunately, I did not consider starting a detoxification protocol at that time.

Years later, when I was in my late 50s, I thought I was completely healthy because I was not taking any prescription medications and did not have any medical conditions. But slowly I started having symptoms indicative of chronic inflammation, including chronic pain or discomfort in the joints of both hands, early erectile dysfunction, and mildly decreased urinary stream. In addition, an old chronic traumatic injury to my left hip pain was getting worse, slowly but steadily. Denial is a powerful coping mechanism, and I attributed my hand discomfort to doing too many colonoscopies, the decreased urinary stream and erectile dysfunction to the normal aging process, etc. But now my blood pressure systolic, which traditionally had been in the 110s and 120s increased to the 130s. I checked a few fasting blood sugars and they were "normal" in the 90's but already higher than ideal, which is 86 or lower. The final straw that broke the camel's back was when I came home from a restaurant and checked a 2-hour post meal blood glucose. It was 140, which is the lowest number to diagnose prediabetes. Although that restaurant meal had plenty of carbohydrates (pizza), it was the only dish I ate, no desert that day. In order to find out my glucose over the prior three months I did an A1c. It was 5.7, the lowest number that is considered prediabetes, and this finally got me out of my denial state. For many years I had been given my patients my health guidelines. Now it was the time for me to also follow my own guidelines, which eventually become the book *Fountain of Health. Regain your Health, Happiness and lose Weight. A revolution in Health for everybody*, which I followed very carefully.

Many thousands of glucose testing were involved to come up with these guidelines. All symptoms improved after implementing the 3-hour glucose testing. Although I started with a ketogenic diet, for at least one year, I eventually switched to a relatively high carbohydrate diet just because I enjoy it better. The increased carbohydrate intake did not have any negative effects, probably because I do not eat any refined carbohydrates or any processed food. In addition, I was having a very difficult time keeping an ideal body weight while on a ketogenic diet. Adding more carbohydrates to my diet allow me to gain a few needed pounds of weight, reaching a low normal BMI (body mass index).

During the relatively initial process, I did 5-day fasting (less than 400 calories of vegetables/day) more often, one year I did it eleven times. Now I have decreased 5-day fasting to no more than quarterly.

To my surprise, a big drop in fasting blood glucose happened after taking CDS. Before taking CDS my fasting blood glucose was in the 80's, often in the low 80's but never in the 70's. The initial dose of CDS did not make a difference, but it was the lowest dose recommended of 10 ml

CURE OR PREVENT DIABETES

of CDS in one liter of reverse osmosis water. My fasting glucose improved after increasing CDS to 30-40 ml instead of 10 ml, with fasting glucose even in the high 60s. The benefit happened after taking CDS for a few months. I stopped CDS and eventually my fasting blood glucose returned to the 80's. I can only bring it down to the 70's taking CDS, but the second time only took 2-3 weeks instead of months. The most reasonable explanation is CDS decreased the body's toxin load which benefited the insulin receptor. One fact that greatly encouraged me to try CDS was the huge campaign orchestrated to discredit CDS and Dr. Kalcker. To me, this was a clear indication of big nefarious financial forces at work.

All my previously mentioned signs or symptoms normalized.

SUMMARY OF PERSONAL RESULTS (after implementation of my dietary guidelines).

BLOOD PRESSURE. About four years ago, systolic in the 130's. Now on a non-restricted salt diet, systolic around or below 100. See table.

A1c HEMOGLOBIN. About four years ago, 5.7 (thus, prediabetes). Now 4.7 while eating many carbohydrates (fruits, dried figs, dried apricots, and Medjool dates).

Over the last 3-4 years, the following symptoms were reversed: (a) chronic pain in hand joints, both hands; (b) erectile dysfunction; (c) decreased urinary stream; (d) left hip pain caused by repetitive traumatic injury.

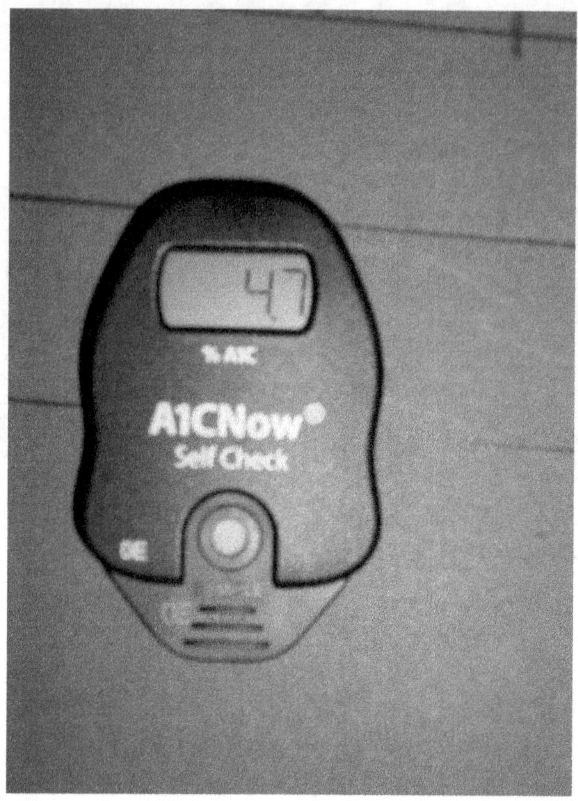

A1c on a non-restricted carbohydrate diet.

BP (blood pressures taking on consecutive days)

SYSTOLIC	DIASTOLIC
85	68
86	69
85	69
93	74
97 (average 101 + 93)	76 (average of 79 + 74)
99	70
99	80
86	69
98	71
99	78
103 (average 108 + 99)	73 (average of 73 + 73)
98	75
90	73
91	75
90	75
99	78
93	70
94	70
91	76
79	65
95	73
98	72
87	69
92	71

AVERAGE:	**AVERAGE:**
92.79	72.45

D. CONCLUSION

Diabetes is reversible unless pancreatic cell damage has already occurred, which usually is a late stage and will make reversal much more difficult.

Insulin resistance can be reversed by using the 3-hour post meal glucose testing at home and avoiding any offending fats. Unhealthy fats should never be ingested, no exceptions to this rule. Healthy fats should not be heated to an unhealthy temperature that will degrade the fats quality. Following the protocol described in this book, it will be possible to improve insulin resistance relatively quickly. This will allow most people to decrease or stop taking diabetic medications. Thus, careful monitoring of blood glucose must be done to avoid hypoglycemic (low blood sugar) episodes.

Curing the insulin receptor is a much more tedious and time-consuming endeavor because detoxification is a slow process. Normalizing the insulin receptor requires extensive detoxification of multiple toxins that have harmed the receptor. Seeking the advice of a functional medicine physician is highly recommended for this detoxification.

Diabetes is a devastating disease which will greatly decrease the quality of life. Every attempt should be made to reverse it. Hopefully this book will be your guiding light.

E. REFERENCES

INTRODUCTION

1. Moran, Manuel. Fountain of Health. Regain your Health, Happiness and lose Weight. A revolution in Health for Everybody. By *Dorrance Publishing* (in print).

CHAPTER 1. DIAGNOSIS

1. Templeman NM, et al. Reduced Circulating Insulin Enhances Insulin Sensitivity in Old Mice and Extends Lifespan. *Cell Reports* 11 July 2017; 20(2): 451-463.

https://reader.elsevier.com/reader/sd/pii/S2211124717308628?token=87E3BFC58BC06B14A26D44 F61797AE549A7ED223340960265A26ECF2B9997C3E26CE05084C1BE7A2D27E5BD633A6C7DB

2. Web based insulin sensitivity calculator.

https://www.thebloodcode.com/homa-ir-calculator/

CHAPTER 2. ETIOLOGY (WHAT CAUSES DIABETES—INSULIN RESISTANCE)

1. Petersen KF, et al. Impaired mitochondrial activity in the insulin-resistant offspring of patients with type 2 diabetes. *N Engl J Med.* 2004 Feb 12; 350(7):664-71.
https://pubmed.ncbi.nlm.nih.gov/14960743/

2. Sweeney S. Dietary factors that influence the dextrose tolerance test. A preliminary study. *Arch Intern Med* 1927; 40(6): 818-830.
https://jamanetwork.com/journals/jamainternalmedicine/fullarticle/535594

3. Krssak M, et al. Intramyocellular lipid concentrations are correlated with insulin sensitivity in humans: a 1H NMR spectroscopy study. *Diabetology* 1999; 42: 113-116.
https://pubmed.ncbi.nlm.nih.gov/10027589/

4. Roden M, et al. Mechanism of Free Fatty Acid-induced insulin Resistance in Humans. *J. Clin. Invest.* 1996; 97: 2859-2865. https://www.ncbi.nlm.nih.gov/pmc/articles/PMC507380/

5. Roden M, Krssak M, Stingl H, et al. Rapid Impairment of Skeletal Muscle Glucose Transport/Phosphorylation by Free Fatty Acids in Humans. *Diabetes* 1999; 48(2): 358-364.
https://link.springer.com/article/10.1023/B:REMD.0000021434.98627.dc

6. Lee S, et al. Effects of an overnight lipid infusion on intramyocellular lipid content and insulin sensitivity in African-American versus Caucasian adolescents. *Metabolism Clinical and Experimental* 2013; 62: 417-423. https://www.metabolismjournal.com/article/S0026-0495(12)00346-0/ppt

7. Santomauro A TMG. Overnight Lowering of Free Fatty Acids With Acipimox Improves Insulin Resistance and Glucose Tolerance in Obese Diabetic and Nondiabetic Subjects. *Diabetes* 1999; 48(9): 1836-41. https://pubmed.ncbi.nlm.nih.gov/10480616/

8. Roden M. How Free Fatty Acids Inhibit Glucose Utilization in Human Skeletal Muscle. *News Physiol Sci* 2004; 19: 92-96. https://pubmed.ncbi.nlm.nih.gov/15143200/

9. Bachmann OP, et al. Effects of Intravenous and Dietary Lipid Challenge on Intramyocellular Lipid Content and the Relation With Insulin Sensitivity in Humans. *Diabetes* 2001; 50: 2579-2584. https://diabetes.diabetesjournals.org/content/50/11/2579

10. Samuel VT, et al. Mechanisms for Insulin Resistance: Common Threads and Missing Links. *Cell* 148, March 2, 2012. https://pubmed.ncbi.nlm.nih.gov/22385956/

11. Rachek LI. Free Fatty Acids and Skeletal Muscle Insulin Resistance. *Progress in Molecular Biology and Translational Science*, Volume 121. https://pubmed.ncbi.nlm.nih.gov/24373240/

12. Evans WJ. Oxygen-Carrying Proteins in Meat and Risk of Diabetes Mellitus. *JAMA Intern Med* 2013; 173(14): 1335-1336. https://pubmed.ncbi.nlm.nih.gov/23778318/

13. Perseghin G, et al. Intramyocellular Triglyceride Content Is a Determinant of in Vivo Insulin Resistance in Humans. *Diabetes* Vol 48, August 1999. 14. Nolan CJ, et al. Lipotoxicity: Why do saturated fatty acids cause and monounsaturated protect against it? *Journal of Gastroenterology and Hepatology* 2009; 24: 703-711. https://diabetes.diabetesjournals.org/content/48/8/1600

15. Ye J. Role of Insulin in the Pathogenesis of Free Fatty Acid-Induced Insulin Resistance in Skeletal Muscle. *Endocrine, Metabolic & Immune Disorders – Drug Targets* 2007; 7: 65-74. https://pubmed.ncbi.nlm.nih.gov/17346204/

16. Estadella D, et al. Lipotoxicity: Effects of Dietary Saturated and Transfatty Acids. *Mediators of Inflammation* 2013; article ID 13. https://www.hindawi.com/journals/mi/2013/137579/

17. Vessby B, et al. Substituting dietary saturated for monounsaturated fat impairs insulin sensitivity in healthy men and women: The KANWU study. *Diabetologia* 2001; 44: 312-319. https://pubmed.ncbi.nlm.nih.gov/11317662/

18. Martins AR, et al. Mechanisms underlying skeletal muscle insulin resistance induced by fatty acids: importance of the mitochondrial function. *Lipids in Health and Disease* 2012; 11: 30. https://pubmed.ncbi.nlm.nih.gov/22360800/

19. Karlic H., et al. Vegetarian Diet Affects Genes of Oxidative Metabolism and Collagen Synthesis. *Annals of Nutrition & Metabolism* 2008; 53: 29-32. https://www.researchgate.net/publication/23238684 Vegetarian Diet Affects Genes of Oxidative Metabolism and Collagen Synthesis

20. Goff LM, et al. Veganism and its relationship with insulin resistance and intramyocellular lipid. *European Journal of Clinical Nutrition* 2005; 59: 291-298. https://pubmed.ncbi.nlm.nih.gov/15523486/

21. Gojda J, et al. Higher insulin sensitivity in vegans is not associated with higher mitochondrial density. *European Journal of Clinical Nutrition* 2013; 1310-1315. https://pubmed.ncbi.nlm.nih.gov/24149445/

22. West KM, et al. Influence of Nutritional Factors on Prevalence of Diabetes. *Diabetes* 1971; 20: 99-108, February. https://diabetes.diabetesjournals.org/content/20/2/99

23. Snowdon DA, et al. Does a Vegetarian Diet Reduce the Occurrence of Diabetes? *Am J Public Health* 1985; 75: 507-512. https://pubmed.ncbi.nlm.nih.gov/3985239/

24. Tonstad S, et al. Vegetarian diets and incidence of diabetes in the Adventist Health Study-2. *Nutrition, Metabolism & Cardiovascular Diseases* 2013; 23: 292-299. https://pubmed.ncbi.nlm.nih.gov/21983060/

25. Chiu THT, et al.   Taiwanese Vegetarians and Omnivores: Dietary Composition, Prevalence of Diabetes and IFG. *PLoS* 2014 February 11; 9(2): e88547.
https://journals.plos.org/plosone/article?id=10.1371/journal.pone.0088547

26. Cunha DA, et al. Death Protein 5 and p53-Upregulated Modulator of Apoptosis Mediate the Endoplasmic Reticulum Stress—Mitochondrial Dialog Triggering Lipotoxic Rodent and Human beta cell Apoptosis. *Diabetes* 2012; 61: 2763-2775.
https://diabetes.diabetesjournals.org/content/61/11/2763.abstract

27. Xiao C, et al. Differential effects of monounsaturated, polyunsaturated and saturated fat ingestion on glucose-stimulated insulin secretion, sensitivity and clearance in overweight and obese, non-diabetic humans.*Diabetologia* 2006; 49: 1371-1379. **(Saturated fat negatively affects insulin secretion and function; increased insulin resistance and decreased insulin production within hours of saturated fat ingestion)** https://pubmed.ncbi.nlm.nih.gov/16596361/

28. Evans WJ. Oxygen-Carrying Proteins in Meat and Risk of Diabetes Mellitus. *JAMA Intern* Med 2013; 173 (14): 1335-1336. **(Red meat consumption increases diabetes risk)**
https://pubmed.ncbi.nlm.nih.gov/23778318/

29. Cao J, Feng XX, Yang NB, et al. Saturated Free Fatty Acid Sodium Palmitate-Induced Lipoapoptosis by Targeting Glycogen Synthase Kinase-3B Activation in Human Liver Cells. *Dig Dis Sci* 2014; February 59(2): 346-57 **(Fat—e.g., palmitate-- in meat and dairy are universally toxic; fat in nuts and avocados (monounsaturated fatty acids—MUFA—e.g., oleat—are not toxic)**
https://pubmed.ncbi.nlm.nih.gov/24132507/

30. Parker DR, et al. Relationship of dietary saturated fatty acids and body habitus to serum insulin concentrations: the Normative Aging Study. *Am J Clin Nutr* 1993; 58: 129-36. **(Obesity and saturated fat intake increase fasting and postprandrial insulin concentrations)**
https://pubmed.ncbi.nlm.nih.gov/8338037/

31. Maron DJ. Saturated Fat Intake and Insulin Resistance in Men With Coronary Artery Disease. *Circulation* 1991; 84: 2020-2027. **(Saturated fat as a contributor to insulin resistance)**
https://pubmed.ncbi.nlm.nih.gov/1934376/

32. Wang L, et al. Plasma fatty acid composition and incidence of diabetes in middle-aged adults: the Atherosclerosis Risk in Communities (ARIC) Study. *Am J Clin Nutr* 2003; 78: 91-8. **(Increased plasma saturated fatty acids increased the risk of diabetes)** https://pubmed.ncbi.nlm.nih.gov/12816776/

33. Taylor R. Pathogenesis of type 2 diabetes: tracing the reverse route from cure to cause. *Diabetologia* 2008; 51: 1781-1789. **(Diabetes is caused by the consumption of too many calories rich in saturated fats in the setting of unfavorable genetic background)** https://pubmed.ncbi.nlm.nih.gov/18726585/

34. Feskens EJ, Sluik D, and Woudenbergh GJ. Meat Consumption, Diabetes, and Its Complications. *Curr Diab Rep* 2013 April; 13(2): 298-306. **(Diabetes risk increased with meat consumption, worse with processed meat and partially for processed poultry)**
https://pubmed.ncbi.nlm.nih.gov/23354681/

35. Palli BB, et al. Association between dietary meat consumption and incident type 2 diabetes: the EPIC-InterAct study. The InterAct Consortium. *Diabetologia* 2013; 56: 47-59. **(Meat consumption increased risk of diabetes; also seen an increase risk of diabetes among workers in the meat industry, unclear cause)** https://pubmed.ncbi.nlm.nih.gov/22983636/

36. Zoncu R, et al. mTor: from growth signal integration to cancer, diabetes and ageing. *Nature Reviews Molecular Biology* January 2011; volume 12. **(Excessive animal/dairy protein/food consumption over stimulates mTor and may increase diabetes due to increase intake of leucine)** https://pubmed.ncbi.nlm.nih.gov/21157483/

37. Liu G, et al. Meat Cooking Methods and Risk of Type 2 Diabetes: Results From Three Prospective Cohort Studies. *Diabetes Care* 2018 Mar; dc171992. **(More diabetes among those cooking their meals at higher temperatures)** https://care.diabetesjournals.org/content/early/2018/03/05/dc17-1992

38. Makhoul Z, Kristal AR, Gulati R, Luick B, Bersamin A, O'Brien D, Hopkins SE, Stephensen CB, Stanhope KL, Havel PJ, Boyer B. **Associations of obesity with triglycerides and C-reactive protein are attenuated in adults with high red blood cell eicosapentaenoic and docosahexaenoic acids**. *European Journal of Clinical Nutrition* 2011; DOI: 10.1038/ejcn.2011.39 https://pubmed.ncbi.nlm.nih.gov/21427737/

39. Hyman MA. Environmental toxins, obesity, and diabetes: an emerging risk factor. *Alternative Therapies;* Mar/April 2010; volume 16, No 2. https://pubmed.ncbi.nlm.nih.gov/20232619/

40. Magliano DJ. Et al. Persistent organic pollutants and diabetes: A review of the epidemiological evidence. *Diabetes & Metabolism* 2014; 40: 1-14. https://pubmed.ncbi.nlm.nih.gov/24262435/

41. Diabetes and the Environment. http://www.diabetesandenvironment.org/home/contam/metals (and https://pubmed.ncbi.nlm.nih.gov/collections/45847237/?sort=pubdate) accessed July 5, 2020.

42. Igbokwe IO, Igwenagu E, and Igbokwe NA. Aluminum toxicosis: a review of toxic actions and effects. *Interdiscip Toxicol* 2019; 12(2): 45-70. Published online 2020 Feb 20. doi: 10.2478/intox-2019-0007 https://www.ncbi.nlm.nih.gov/pmc/articles/PMC7071840/

43. Templeman NM, et al. Reduced Circulating Insulin Enhances Insulin Sensitivity in Old Mice and Extends Lifespan. *Cell Reports* 11 July 2017; 20(2): 451-463. https://pubmed.ncbi.nlm.nih.gov/28700945/

CHAPTER 3. PROBLEM WITH MEDICATIONS THAT INCREASE INSULIN OR WITH INSULIN SUPPLEMENTATION

1. Hong J, Zhang Y, Lai S, Lv A, Su Q, et al. Effects of Metformin Versus Glipizide on Cardiovascular Outcomes in Patients With Type 2 Diabetes and Coronary Artery Disease. *Diabetes Care* 2013; 36(5): 1304-1311. https://care.diabetesjournals.org/content/36/5/1304

2. Goldman MP, Clark CJ, Craven TE, et al. Effect of Intensive Glycemic Control on Risk of Lower Extremity Amputation. *J Am Coll Surg* 2018; 227: 596-604. https://www.journalacs.org/article/S1072-7515(18)32077-5/pdf

CHAPTER 4. 3-HOUR POST-MEAL HOME GLUCOSE TESTING

1. Moran M. Novel protocol for reversing prediabetes and diabetes without medications: The 3-hour post-meal glucose testing. *Int J Complement Alt Med* 2021; 14(1): 1-4.

http://medcraveonline.com/IJCAM/novel-protocol-for-reversing-prediabetes-and-diabetes-without-medications-the-3-hour-post-meal-glucose-testing.html

CHAPTER 5. PROTOCOL FOR REVERSING DIABETES

1. Finnel JS, Saul BC, Goldhamer AC, and Myers TR. Is fasting safe? A chart review of adverse events during medically supervised, water-only fasting. *BMC Complement Altern Med* 2018; 18: 67. https://www.ncbi.nlm.nih.gov/pmc/articles/PMC5819235/

2. Fung TT et al. Low-carbohydrate diets and all-cause and cause-specific mortality: two cohort studies. *Ann Intern Med.* 2010 Sep 7;153(5):289-98. doi: 10.7326/0003-4819-153-5-201009070-00003. https://www.ncbi.nlm.nih.gov/pubmed/?term=Ann+Intern+Med.+2010%3B+153%3A289

3. Chiu THT, et al.   Taiwanese Vegetarians and Omnivores: Dietary Composition, Prevalence of Diabetes and IFG. *PLoS* 2014 February 11; 9(2): e88547. https://pubmed.ncbi.nlm.nih.gov/24523914/

4. Snowdon DA, et al. Does a Vegetarian Diet Reduce the Occurrence of Diabetes? *Am J Public Health* 1985; 75: 507-512. https://pubmed.ncbi.nlm.nih.gov/3985239/

5. Levine ME, et al. Low protein intake is associated with a major reduction in IGF-1, cancer, and overall mortality in the 65 and younger but not older population. *Cell Metab.* 2014 Mar 4;19(3):407-17. doi: 10.1016/j.cmet.2014.02.006. https://www.nih.gov/news-events/nih-research-matters/protein-consumption-linked-longevity and https://www.ncbi.nlm.nih.gov/pubmed/24606898

CHAPTER 6. ETIOLOGY (WHAT HARMS THE INSULIN RECEPTOR).

1. Lee D-H, Lee I-K, Song K, Steffes M, Toscano W, Baker BA, and Jacobs DR. A Strong Dose-Respondent Relation Between Serum Concentrations of Persistent Organic Pollutants and Diabetes. *Diabetes Care* 2006; 29: 1638-1644. https://pubmed.ncbi.nlm.nih.gov/16801591/

2. Pizzorny J. Is the Diabetes Epidemic Primarily Due to Toxins? *Integrative Medicine* 2016; 15(4): 8-17. https://pubmed.ncbi.nlm.nih.gov/27574488/